HOW TO FIGHT THE CRIPPLING PAIN OF PERIPHERAL ARTERIAL DISEASE

SELF HELP GUIDE TO IMPROVE BLOOD FLOW

KEVIN THOMAS MORGAN

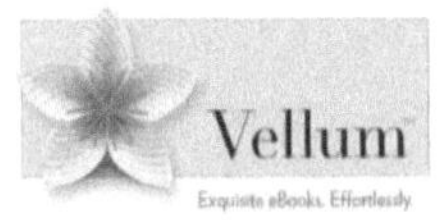

COVER IMAGE

The author with his support crew, Tracey, after he won his age group, 75-79, at the 2022, Wilmington Half Ironman race, NC, USA.

I dedicate this book to a remarkable person, Kymberlie McNicholas, who fights daily to help vascular patients avoid unnecessary peripheral arterial disease (PAD)-related amputations, while teaching them how to get on with their lives.

MEDICAL DISCLAIMER

Medical Disclaimer

This work is no substitute for professional medical advice and treatment. However, once you leave the doctor's office or the operating room you have to work out how to live your life. This book explains how the author addresses his vascular challenges, which include an abdominal aortic aneurysm (AAA) and progressive peripheral arterial disease (PAD). Both have a genetic basis in his case. Dr. Morgan does have the advantage of medical training, as a veterinary pathologist and researcher. The author does not provide medical advice to human animals. If you undertake or modify an exercise program, consult your medical advisors before doing so. Undertaking activities pursued by the author does not mean that he endorses others undertaking such activities, which is clearly their decision and responsibility.

Be careful and sensible, please.

FitOldDog, Old Dogs in Training, LLC

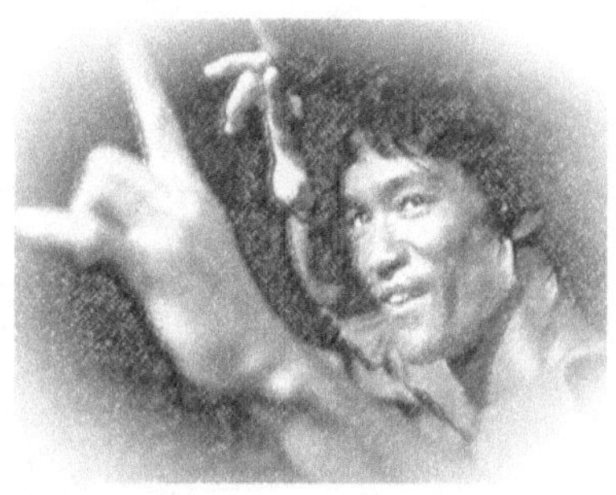

Are you going to let the obstacles in your life be stumbling blocks or stepping stones?

— Bruce Lee

ABOUT THIS BOOK

*"Peripheral arterial disease (PAD) in the legs or lower
extremities, is the narrowing or blockage of the vessels that
carry blood from the heart to the legs. It is primarily caused
by the build-up of fatty plaque in the arteries, which is called
atherosclerosis. PAD can happen in any blood vessel, but it is
more common in the legs than the arms."*

— CDC website, Nov., 2022

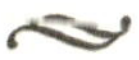

The approach I use to fight this crippling condition is
no substitute for an experienced vascular surgery team.
My symptoms are confined to my calves and feet, which
defines the limits of my personal experience. As a life-
long athlete and student of body movement, with

veterinary medical training, my approaches are based on the anatomy and physiology of the cardiovascular, musculoskeletal, nervous, and other body systems.

I cannot capture every PAD patient's experience, as there is a wide spectrum of location and severity of symptoms. The purpose of this book is to provide fellow PAD sufferers with some personal control over their life, using concepts and techniques I developed over the last seven-years. Each of the approaches outlined improved my ability to walk and run, while permitting my continued enjoyment of Ironman Triathlons.

Most importantly, this work has helped me to master the despair that can accompany the physical challenges associated with this condition. You don't have to have PAD to benefit from reading this book. Based on prevalence data, especially as we age, you may well be needed to step in and provide support to a loved one with this horrible disease.

Please don't hesitate to send any questions, or suggestions for improvements to the book to *olddogin-training@gmail.com*. You can also sign up for my weekly newsletter if you so desire, via *athletewithstent.com*.

Keep moving, whatever you do.

Dr. Kevin Thomas Morgan, BVSc, PhD, DipACVP, FRCPath

PS Thank you Kym, for this attractive award.

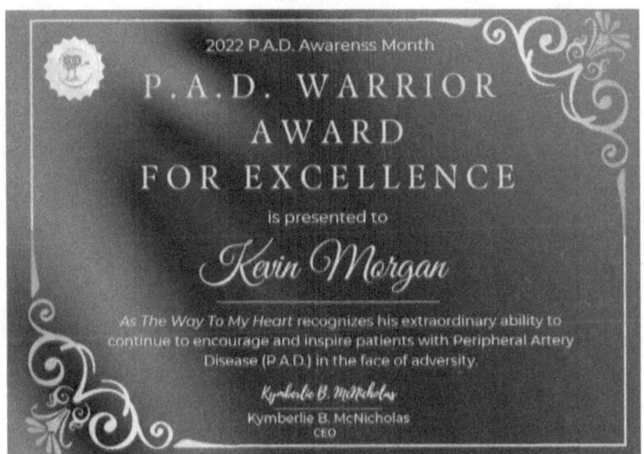

INTRODUCTION

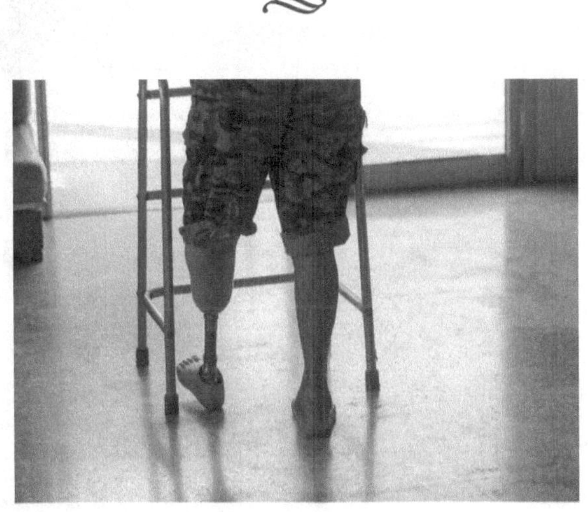

Each year, more than 150,000 amputations are performed in the US to remove toes, legs or feet affected by advanced peripheral artery disease (PAD). Modern treatment options

can restore blood flow to affected limbs and reduce the risk of amputation.

— Coastal Vascular Center, Nov 14, 2022, Peripheral Vascular Disease

PAD is a Plumbing Problem

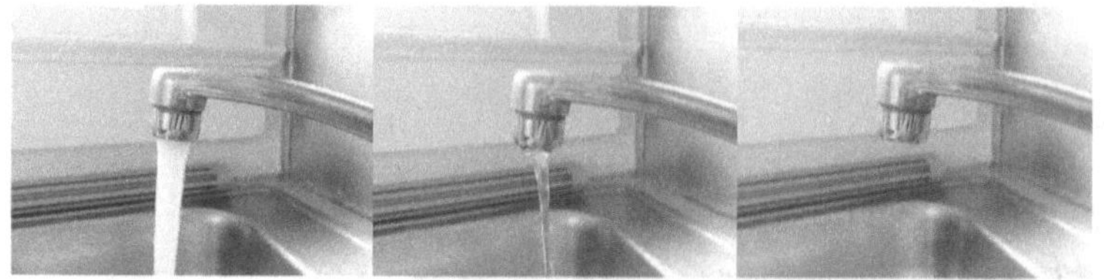

Narrow the pipe, increase resistance, slow the flow.

Fortunately, our bodies can grow new vessels to carry blood around the blockage. These are known as collaterals. Exercise, including walking, encourages their growth.

While these collaterals are growing our bodies apparently attempt to force blood past the blockage by increasing blood pressure. Now we have hypertension as well as PAD. This leads to other problems, such as damage to our eyes and kidneys. This is why doctors prescribe pills designed to bring down our excessively high blood pressure.

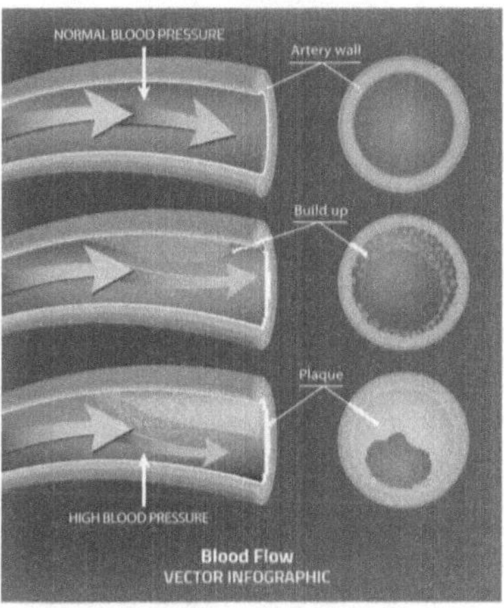

Our body apparently attempts to force blood past the blockage by increasing our blood pressure.

Blood pressure pills can correct our hypertension but they do nothing to help blood flow through blocked arteries. In fact, they reduce the flow. Furthermore, some blood pressure treatments such as beta-blockers, prevent us from increasing our heart rate. This interferes with our ability to exercise, plus they have some nasty side effects, including vertigo (loss of balance).

Exercise is an important way to strengthen our bodies, so we can earn a living and to have some fun.

I encounter PAD, damn!

In 2014 I started to develop numb feet during long runs. By long runs, I mean 26.2-mile marathons. This was soon followed by exercise-induced calf pain in my right leg which severely interfered with running. It even gave me trouble walking uphill.

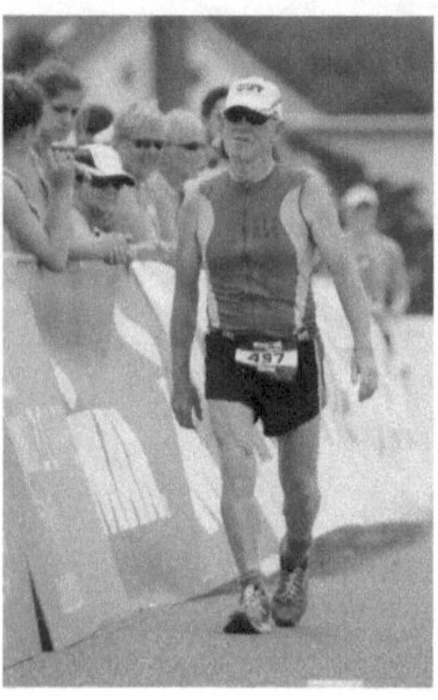

Foot numbness ruined that race in 2014.

My vascular surgeon, Mark, has saved my life from an abdominal aortic aneurysm (AAA) several times since it was found in 2010. I was lucky it didn't kill me. Your aorta is the largest artery in your body, and if it breaks you're dead in no time. Mark's team installed an AAA stent graft to prevent this unfortunate eventuality.

In 2015, they ran a routine Ankle Brachial Index (ABI) Pressure test as part of my annual AAA stent checkup. They look for leaks and other problems. After the ABI test Mark informed me that I'd developed significant PAD.

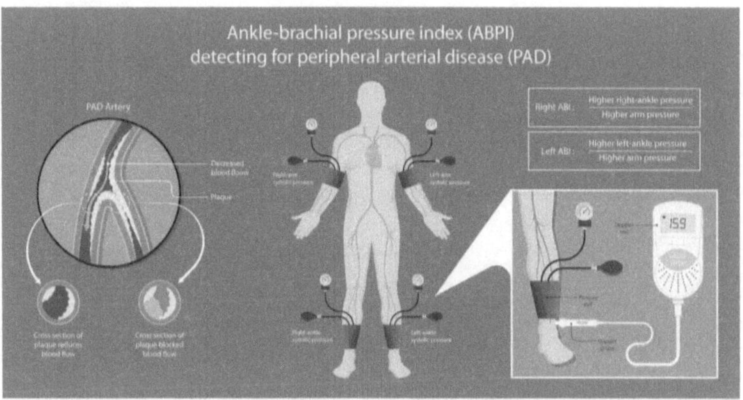

The ABI test used to diagnose PAD.

He said my numb feet and calf pain were a consequence of blockage of the popliteal arteries in my legs as a result of atherosclerosis. Mark also said with a hint of doom that this disease is progressive. I wasn't unduly surprised as I'd known since my early 30s that I have genetically high fat levels in my blood (*dyslipidemia*). This is a common cause of atherosclerosis.

I asked Mark about possible surgical interventions in the form of angioplasty (balloon to open up the arteries) or a stent (a plastic and metal tube inserted into arteries to keep them open). He recommended against surgery in my case, saying, *"Kevin, I could do that, but you need to know that you may lose your leg in the process."*

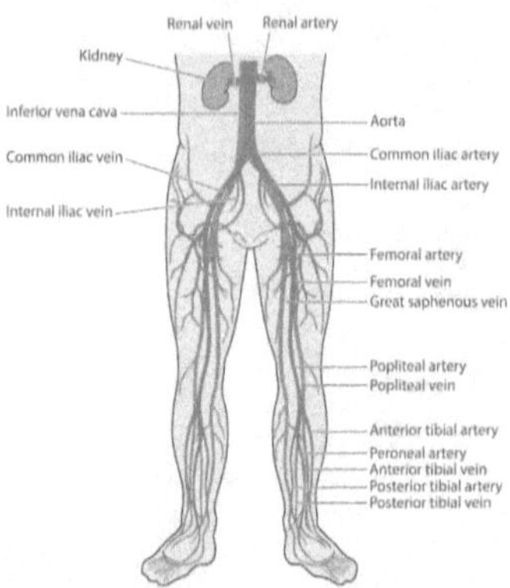

*A little Anatomy goes a long way toward understanding
and fighting PAD. Really no big deal once you get past
the funny names. It's just plumbing, after all.*

As an alternative Mark suggested I undertake a walking program of three thirty-minute walks per week to encourage the growth of collaterals around my blocked popliteal arteries. I remember thinking, *"I'll be doing more than three walks a week."* But surgeons are busy saving people's lives. They don't have time for my chit chat so I kept mum, thinking, *"I'll write a book about it, if I'm successful."*

This is that book!

I thanked Mark for his trouble, and two weeks later struggled through yet another nightmarish marathon. With numb feet and a painful right calf I stumbled over the finish line just as they were closing the course. This was a far cry from my running in the Boston Marathon, in 2009.

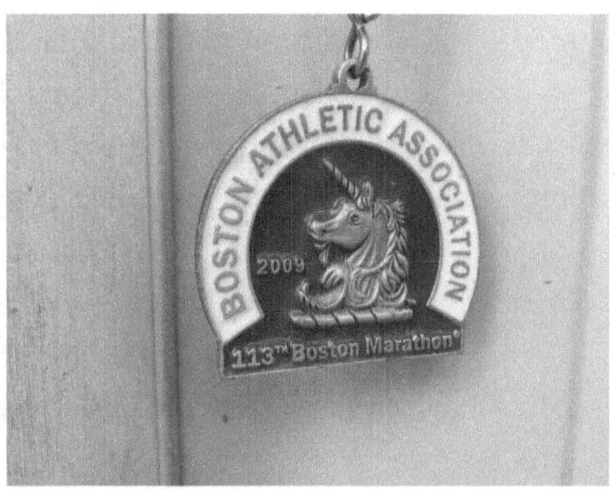

After discovering my AAA in 2010 I successfully continued Ironman training by making modifications to protect my AAA stent graft. With this in mind in 2015, in Mark's consulting room, I decided to find a way to continue Ironman with PAD. Though less lethal than an AAA, PAD is more horrible! The AAA breaks and you're dead. PAD delivers endless pain, incapacity, and often loss of toes, feet, even legs.

A challenge worthy of a veterinary pathologist and Ironman distance triathlete don't you think? Then a movie came to mind.

The Martian

Due to a storm and an accident, astronaut and botanist *Mark Watney* is marooned on a desolate planet, Mars. He can't be rescued by NASA for several years. He has life support and essential supplies designed to last him and his prematurely departed five-member crew for a few months. At first he's dejected and feels sorry for himself. In case he dies, which is highly likely, Mark decides to record a video diary. During one recording he looks at his image on the screen and says to himself,

"I'm going to have to science the shit out of this."

Mark looks immediately more upbeat. He's going to take control of an insurmountable task, surviving on Mars for years. Later, after another life-threatening disaster beyond his control, you see Mark start to give into despair, again. But he rebounds, saying, *"F*ck you, Mars."*

I've said the same to PAD.

There are so many important messages in that movie for us PAD sufferers, and for humans swamping planet Earth, depleting our resources. Mark comes to appreciate the potatoes he manages to grow in his own excrement, and which save his life. I am reminded of that scene each time the first shoots arrive in my vegetable garden.

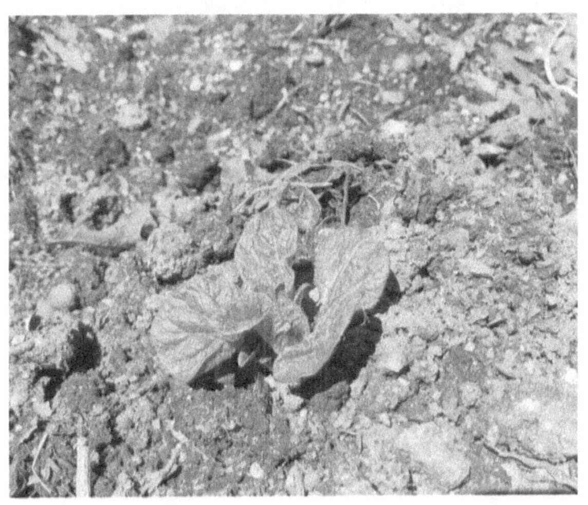

This always seems like magic.

After receiving the AAA stent graft, in 2010, I asked my surgeon, Joe, what he thought about my ability to continue Ironman training. He looked at me with an odd expression, and said, *"If I were you, I'd go easy at first."*

Instead of going easy, once the surgery site was healed, I decided to work out how to continue my training. The following year I managed to finish the Lake Placid Ironman with my AAA stent graft.

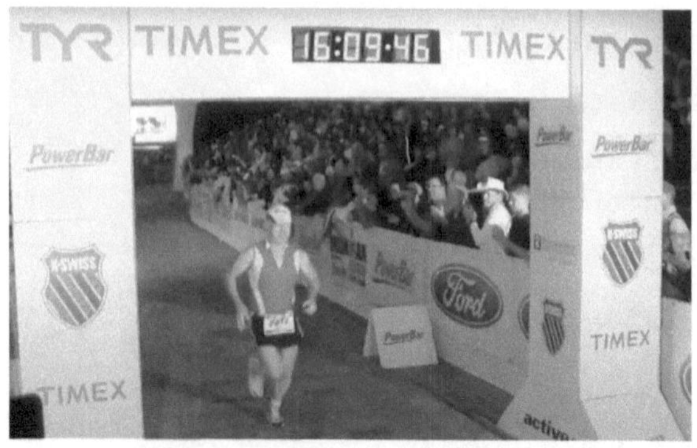

*I finished the 2011 Lake Placid Ironman with an AAA
stent graft, so why not with PAD?*

When it comes to PAD, some days I feel like giving up. The calf pain when I run can be horrible. The thought passes through my mind, *"Why don't you accept your age, Kevin? Have a glass of wine and chill out."*

This thought immediately evaporates to be replaced by *"No f-ing way! Mark Watney did it so why not me?"* Excuse my French as we say in the UK. Furthermore, I'm a pathologist not a botanist, which is more useful for fighting PAD, but not for growing potatoes on Mars.

Pathology is a branch of medical science that involves the study and diagnosis of disease.

— Pathology Department, McGill University

After a little research and lots of reflection I developed four angles of attack on my blocked popliteal arteries problem:

1. Improve blood flow to my feet.
2. Reduce flow resistance in my feet.
3. Aid venous return from my feet.
4. Maintain my optimism on those rare bad days.

PAD is a humdinger of a disease. I do have occasional bad days when the task feels overwhelming, Ironman or no Ironman. I just say to myself, *"F*ck you, PAD."*

Over the last seven years I've tested one movement modification after another. I assessed each for its contribution to my walking and running. By the way, my PAD has little or no impact on swimming or cycling, except during steep hill climbs on the bike when I get a little calf tightness. The changes I made are the basis of the 12-step program in this book.

Why it turned out to be 12 steps I've no idea.

Maybe 12 steps is a self-help universal constant, like those magical numbers, "Pi" and "e," who knows?

As you can imagine, I'd like to keep my feet for as long as possible, and to help you keep yours. I also wish to continue Ironman-distance triathlons, which consist of a 2.4-mile open-water swim, a 112-mile bike ride and a full 26.2-mile marathon run, all in one day.

People say I'm crazy to do it at age 79. But I love it!

Important Note: You don't have to do Ironman or be any kind of athlete to do the work outlined in this book. It would be best if you employ physical activities that you enjoy, and I strongly recommend a walking program. Maybe you could add a little science in there too? It's all over the place.

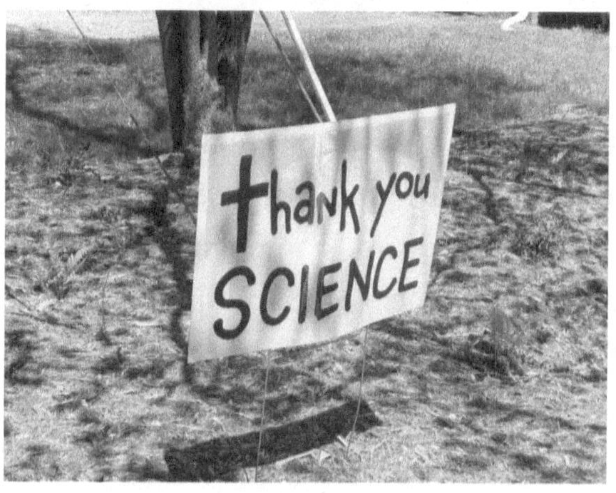

Thanks, Mum, for enabling my science education.

A Brief Note On Pain

Before reaching for pain killers please remember that pain is designed to protect you from further harm. Think of a kid touching a hot stove. Only happens once. A person with leprosy would touch the hot stove and have no idea, allowing for further damage. Your body is saying with its pain response, *"Do something for heaven's sake."*

Claudication is pain caused by too little blood flow to muscles during exercise. Most often this pain occurs in the legs after walking at a certain pace and for a certain amount of time — depending on the severity of the condition.

— Mayo Clinic

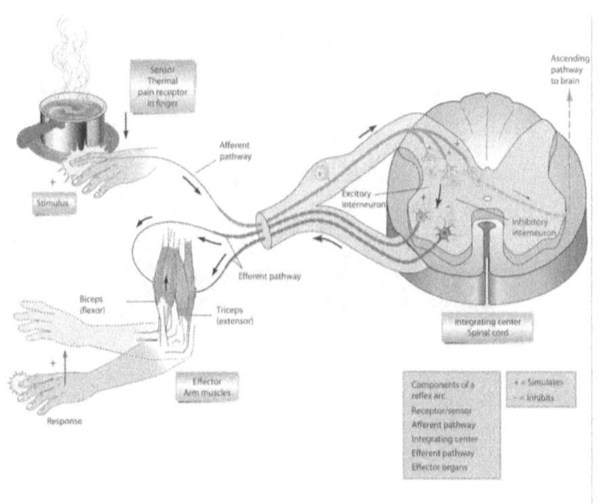

The pain reflex protection circuit.

Loss of blood supply due to atherosclerosis can lead to life-threatening gangrene. Thank goodness for claudication. I see pain as my teacher and while running as my coach. Pain is my body's way of saying, *"Watch your pace, Kevin. Soften those feet and spread those toes, Kevin. What the hell are you doing, Kevin?"*

Here's a recent example of an intense foot pain that provided me with some running instruction.

As I went through the finish chute of the 2022

NC70.3 Half Ironman race, the ball of my right foot was on fire. I wondered what the hell was going on.

I finished in spite of the pain, which earned me a spot in the 2023 World Half Ironman Championships in Finland. There were only 17 of those coveted slots for a field of 3,000 athletes and I got one by finishing first in my age-group.

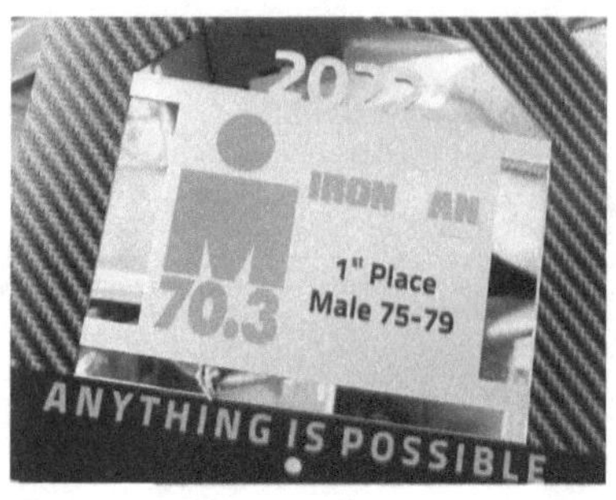

Luck of the devil, some say.

I finished in spite of the pain, I reply.

The next morning I found several small corns on the ball of my right foot. One near my big toe and two near the little one.

Corns and calluses are thick, hardened layers of skin that develop when the skin tries to protect itself against friction or pressure. They often form on feet and toes or hands and fingers. For most people, simply removing the source of the friction or pressure makes corns and calluses disappear.

— Mayo Clinic

The key phrase: "... *simply removing the source of the friction or pressure ...*"

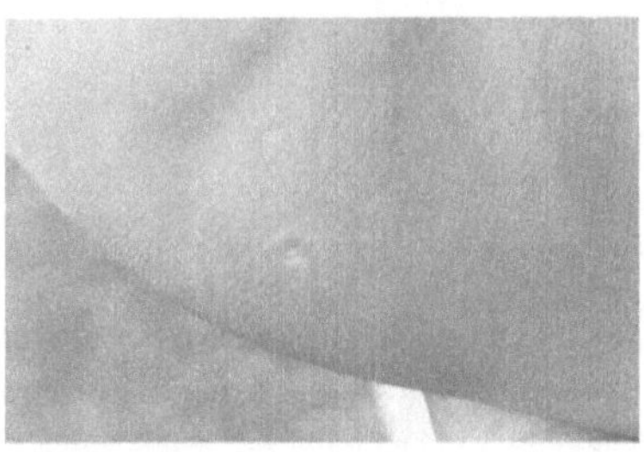

Those corns don't look much but they hurt like hell if you upset them.

We lose fat padding on the soles of our feet as we age, and I'm approaching 80. Bummer! This loss of fat is called *Fat Pad Atrophy*. Great! Now I'm atrophying.

Those corns were a consequence of poor foot mechanics, due to an inadequate blood supply, combined with age-related fat atrophy. Loss of padding would expose the metatarsal-phalangeal joint regions in the ball of my feet to impact and pressure stress.

*"Here we go! Another problem to science the sh*t out of! And a tough one, too! I have to optimize my foot mechanics in the face of a suboptimal blood supply to the very muscles that operate my foot mechanics?"*

THE ANKLE JOINT IN SIDE VIEW

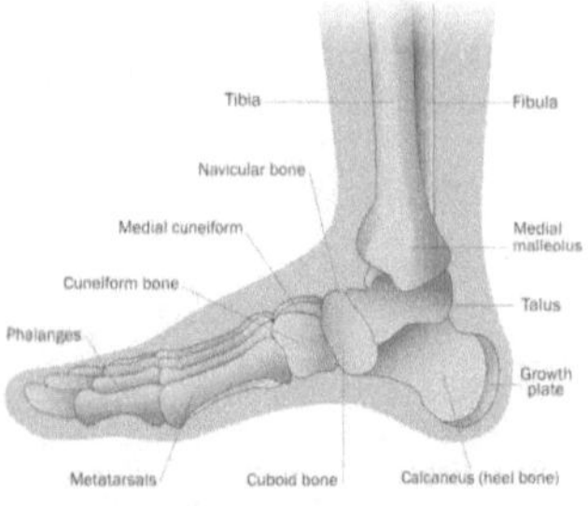

Note how the metatarsal-phalangeal joints, at the base of the toes, are close to the ground, exposing them to impact stresses, which would be made worse by fat atrophy.

Of course, I'm using the methods described in this book. As they say, *"Physician, heal thyself!"*

My corns are slowly fading as I apply steps 1, 2, 8 and 9, plus this other trick I developed. In order to take the impact stresses away from where the corns reside, I imagine putting the load on my middle toe. This is a mind game aided by my previous work to control my toes individually. I finally stopped wearing sock, and the corns faded away.

I see corns as my foot mechanics coaches. They tell me when I'm putting undue stress on that lateral metatarsal-phalangeal joint region. They are like my old martial arts coaches who administered pain if they thought we weren't trying hard enough. It worked amazingly well, as do those bloody corns.

Thanks for the great coaching, corns!

Can't do much about fat atrophy, except maybe gel inserts in my running shoes. Yet to find inserts that work but I may be forced to find some eventually.

When I make changes to my walking or running, I first test them on a treadmill. Treadmills, which are easier on our feet, enable better control of foot mechanics. Once I have whatever it is working on the treadmill, I move outside to the *asphalt* road. I never run on concrete if it can be avoided. It's too unforgiving a surface for my feet. If all is well on the road, I then test my new techniques at local running races.

Optimizing foot mechanics and other aspects of walking and running with PAD is a slowly progressive process. It's certainly worth the effort! I ran a local 8k race the other day, as part of this work, where my little dog, Gizmo, and I had a great time. He slept so well, afterwards.

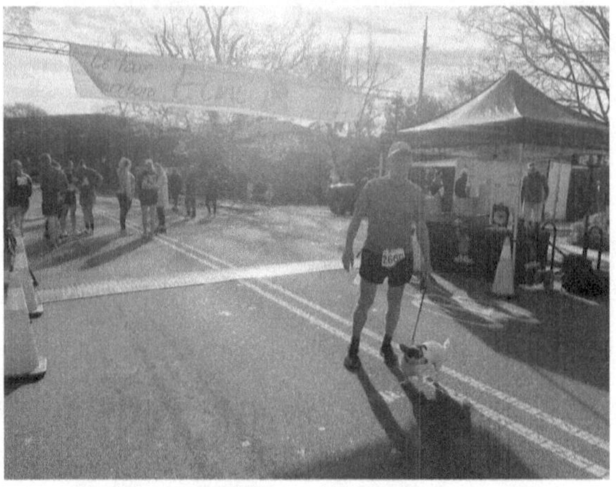

At the finish line of the 2022 Carrboro Gallop &
Gorge 8k Thanksgiving race with Gizmo. A tired but
happy little chap.

A final warning:

I'm talking about quite a bit of training. You need to realize the amount of work one does to be fit enough for Ironman. I'm sure this training has helped me. For instance, here is one of the training rides I completed prior to my latest half Ironman, the one that has me going to Finland next year.

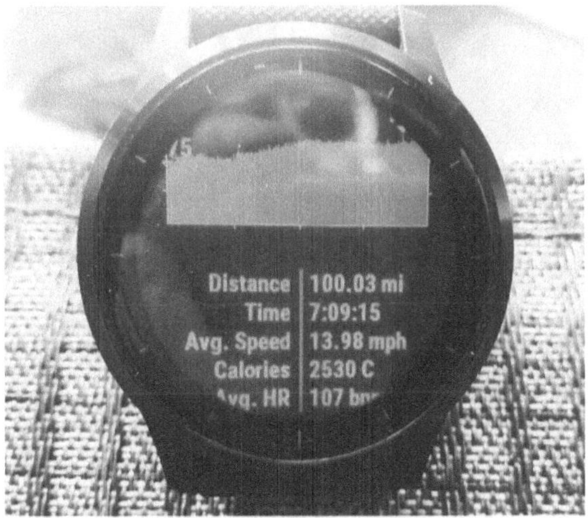

PAD is serious!

We have to be equally serious in our work to beat it.

Take a deep breath!

Now let's get you started.

1

STEP ONE: SPREAD YOUR FEET

Spread your toes and get to know your feet.

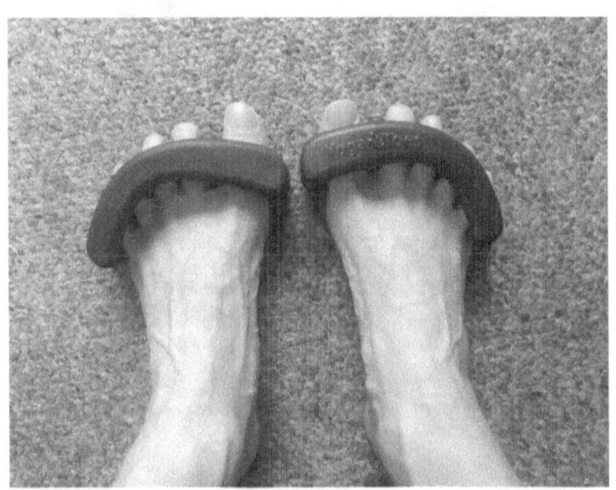

*My Yoga Toes® sure are helping blood flow through
my feet.*

Spreading your feet is the opposite of scrunching them up, and fortunately there is a way to do this. With Yoga Toes®! You can use your fingers to spread your toes but it's harder to do. I found that spreading my toes dramatically improved foot mechanics, helping me to share the load across the balls of my feet. Young or old, Yoga Toes® really help our feet, when used appropriately *(I have no financial interest).*

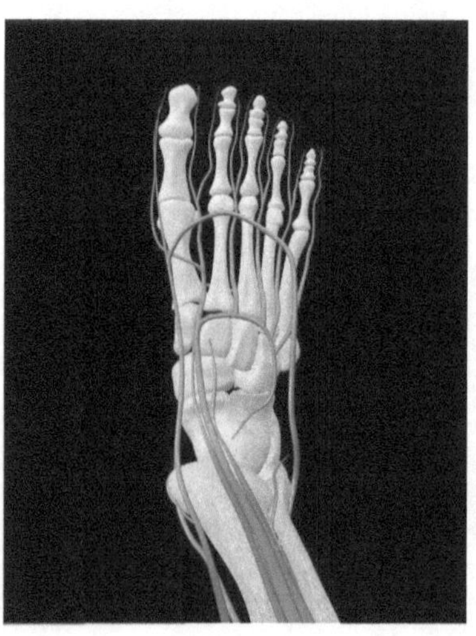

Bones and blood vessels of the foot. Notice how certain vessels lie between the metatarsal bones.

Widening my feet using Yoga Toes® dramatically delays the onset of claudication when I run, and it has eliminated foot numbness, as I walk uphill or run, due to better blood flow through my feet. Spreading my toes separates those long bones in my feet, the metatarsals. This would reduce compression of blood vessels that lie between those metatarsals, to reduce resistance to blood flow.

Furthermore, activation of my toes improved the conversation between my feet and the ground, which enhances the massaging of blood, and other tissue fluids, through my feet.

These tools are great, but don't go crazy at first. *Little and often is the trick.* You don't want to irritate your feet by doing too much too soon. Start with a few sessions of several minutes a day, working up to 2 x 20 minutes or more.

The use of Yoga toes® is nicely demonstrated in a short video on the FitOldDog YouTube channel, entitled *"An Introductory Lesson On Yoga Toes by Rebecca, FitOldDog's Continuum and Dance Teacher."*

I noticed that we made that video 12 years ago. It has over 25,000 views, 85 positive reviews, and no negative reviews. This means our work is helping people. Rebecca taught me so much about healthy movement, she even fixed my horrible posture.

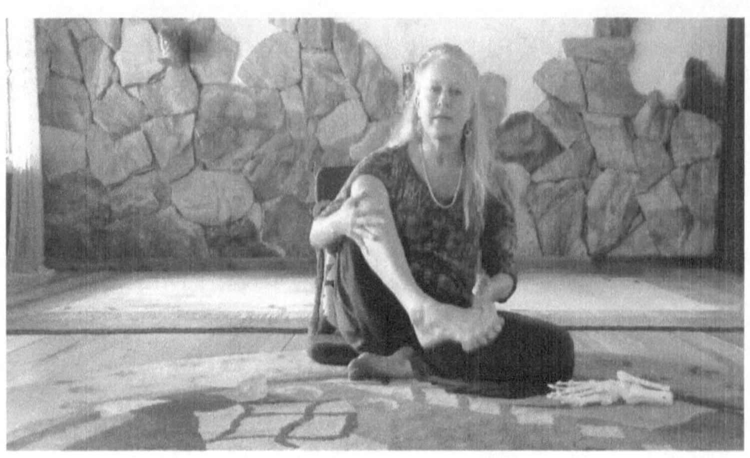

Rebecca does a great job of explaining things.

Get to know your feet and start spreading those toes and metatarsals, and move on to Step Two.

2

STEP TWO: SOFTEN YOUR FEET

Soft feet reduce flow resistance.

Here's a simple demonstration of the way in which fluids penetrate more freely through uncompressed tissues.

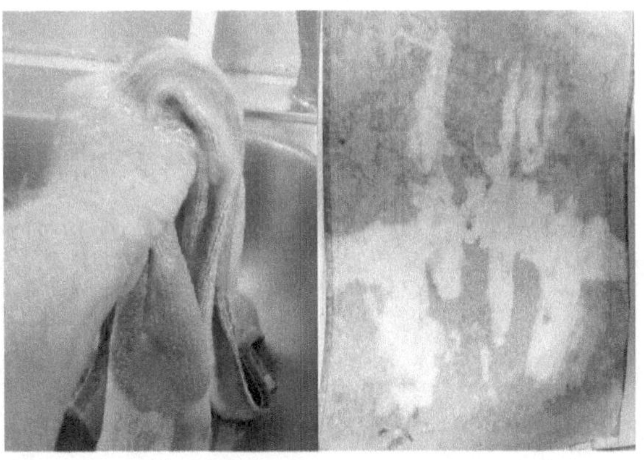

My dish towel demonstration of compression inhibiting fluid flow.

(Left) I rolled an old dish towel lengthwise, gently squeezed the middle in my fist and proceeded to soak the towel under a kitchen tap for several minutes.

(Right) I then unrolled the towel onto the counter, to reveal that the compressed region was completely dry (white) while the rest of the towel was soaking wet (gray).

Compression of your feet by tight shoes, tube socks, or gripping in response to pain, will inhibit penetration of blood into and through your feet. This will resist arterial flow into your foot due to back pressure. It will also inhibit venous return "downstream," by impairing blood delivery to your venous system on its way back to your heart.

All due to compressing your feet.

Back pressure:
Opposition to flow of a liquid or gas due to friction, inertia, gravity, or other cause.

— Merriam Webster Online Dictionary

Thus the need for soft, wide, relaxed feet, even in the face of calf and foot pain. Think like a plumber.

Developing soft-feet is a mind game.

Your feet might be soft, but they are not passively

soft, as you walk or run. They are carrying out an intense conversation with the ground. This they do through input from thousands of receptors on the soles of your feet that send signals to your spinal cord and brain. This information is then used to fine-tune the activity of muscles in your feet, around your ankles and calves, and throughout your body.

Some magic trick, don't you think? Impresses the hell out of me whenever I think about it.

There are literally thousands of receptors for pressure, vibration, temperature, and so forth, embedded in the soles of your feet. All of this is integrated with your location and balance systems.

Try saying to your feet, out loud as you walk, *"Soft feet, please."* No one else is listening or cares but your feet will hear you. They care a lot. People forget that their feet are very much alive. It's also important to be kind to your feet at home. Ironman isn't very kind to my feet which is why I treated myself to these soft sexy slippers.

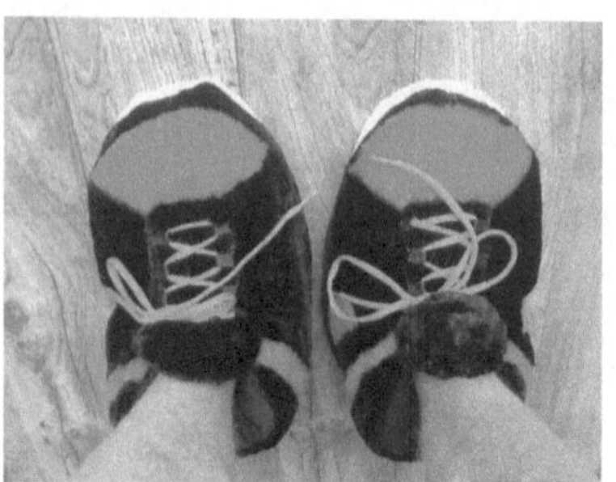

It's important to be kind to your feet.

3

STEP THREE: USE THE BEST SOCKS AND SHOES

Wear the right shoes and socks so your soft feet can spread and talk clearly to the ground.

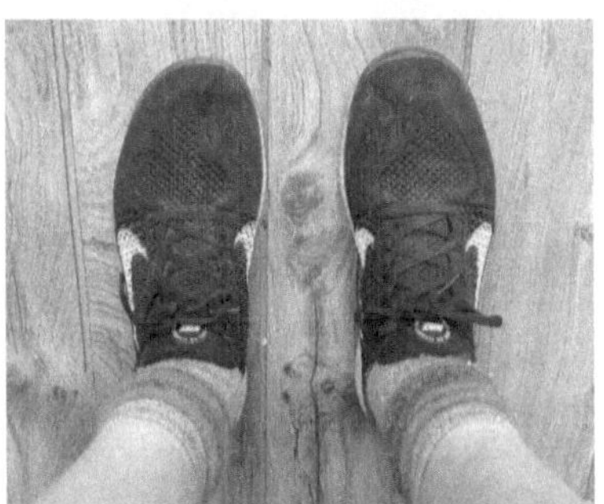

I'm no shoe expert and I won't promote particular brands. I use minimalist shoes with thick wool socks. For you, the proof of the pudding will be in the eating, as they say.

Choice of shoes and socks for walking or running with PAD is a fascinating and important topic. Finding your optimal footwear requires experimentation and, as for all things PAD, it requires patience and awareness. Whatever footwear you choose it is essential that they permit your feet to spread, relax, and talk to the ground.

Your feet, legs and hips will let you know what works. The message may be deceptive. Sometimes a foot problem leads to pain in the form of a tight hip or a painful shoulder muscle. Decoding these messages can be tricky because the perceived location of pain isn't always where the problem lies.

I suspect our feet are more intelligent than we are, so it pays to pay attention to what they have to say.

Socks

You need socks that protect your feet from abrasions, while optimizing the flow of blood into, through, and out of your feet. Socks with tight ankles will compress tissues around arteries and veins reducing flow. Tube socks, unless you have thin feet, squeeze the foot laterally, compressing blood vessels that lie between the metatarsal bones.

Conclusion: I don't like tube socks or any footwear that compresses or restrains the freedom of my feet.

Furthermore, I have somewhat frail skin. This makes sense as I have an aortic aneurysm due to a connective tissue weakness, thus my preference for thick, woolen protective socks, and the lanolin in wool is good for my feet, too!

You will have to work out what works for you, but don't worry, your feet will let you know if they don't like your choices.

Shoes

My basic guidelines for shoes include a wide toe box so your feet can spread. You may consult a podiatrist or sports medicine doctor, but it's your feet that should make the final call.

For long walks on rough terrain or during stormy weather I wear sturdy, comfortable-fitting hiking shoes. The rest of the time I stick to my minimalist running shoes. These are basically a flat piece of rubber compound that protects the soles of my feet. No thick heel or builtin supports for pronation or supination! They are nothing like the "regular" running shoes most people wear, which are more like orthotics in my opinion. Beware the shoe industry taking you down an expensive footwear rabbit hole. Listen to your feet instead.

Minimalist shoes do place a tremendous load on my feet, which have to be strong, flexible, intelligent, and well conditioned for the tasks they undertake. Intelligent? Sure! My feet have to work with the terrain to which they "talk" physically. Walking and running involve a complex conversation between your whole body and road, with your feet acting as skilled interpreters.

4

———

STEP FOUR: EMPLOY YOUR WHOLE BODY

Read Jack Heggie's great book, do the exercises, and everything will change for the better when walking or running.

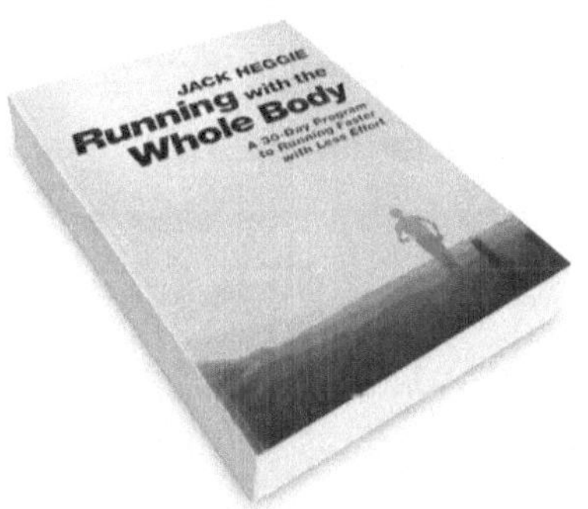

This book was recommended to me by a great Physical Therapist (PT). Thanks, Bruce.

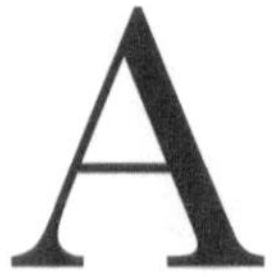walk in the park with PAD is no walk in the park. Always makes me laugh when I think of that linguistic paradox.

Learning how to walk with your whole body is a critical skill for your battle against PAD. If you buy Jack Heggie's book (in which, again, I have no financial interest) and do the exercises you will be on your way to incorporating the magic of Feldenkrais into your life. Whole body walking begins with effective shoulder-hip counter rotation. As your right shoulder comes forward your right hip goes back. This will cause your feet to come in more gently, from the outside edge, rather than heel striking.

Whole body walking is a skill you will need to master. It is easy once you get the feel for it.

Walking is a critical activity for the creation of those all-important collaterals. You could even join a walking group to keep your training on track.

When my PAD came on in earnest my right calf would lock up painfully, especially at the beginning of the walk or when walking uphill. I'd have to stop frequently to take weight off my right foot so that calf could fill with blood. This refill process hurt a bunch. After developing the approaches described in this book, I rarely have to stop, even when walking hills or running, as long as I don't push it too hard.

Pace is critical!

As a runner I know the first mile is always the worst mile, PAD or no PAD. This is also true for walking with PAD, which is why you have to persist past that first mile.

Important: you cannot judge how well you will do at the beginning of a walk or run, or based on how you feel before you start. Exercise is funny that way. I've had some of my best workouts when I didn't want to train, and some of the worst when I started out gung ho.

I think collateral blood vessels like to close up when not in use, and take a while to open up when you get moving. Think about it! They aren't really meant to be there in the first place. I used to find that it took at least a mile or two of walking or running before claudication pain started to fade. After doing the work described, I can now walk claudication free for miles, if I get my pace right. Even my walking and running pace are becoming faster.

Running is much harder than walking. I have to ease into it more slowly than I did when I was younger. Since doing the work explained in this book, I no longer have to stop in the way I describe in my book on training for aging. It was pretty depressing at the time, as you can tell from what I wrote three years ago.

"We run 100 yards, 200 yards, 250, and then we stop. I stand immobile on my left leg, as pain surges through my right calf. Willbe [my yellow lab] sits patiently at my side. He knows the drill. I glance at my watch as it calculates

average running pace. It grows from 9 minutes and 30 seconds per mile, through 10 minutes, 11 minutes and finally 18 minutes and 20 seconds per mile. This is not much better than a brisk walking pace."

Time was moving, while we were not!

No more! Here's a recording from one of my recent three-mile runs:

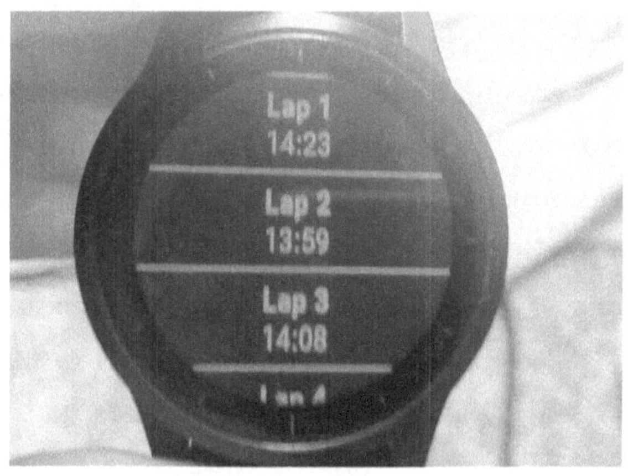

I'm working toward a goal of 12-minute mile pace.
One can dream.

You will benefit from whole-body low impact walking in other ways. If your heels are the first to hit the ground (heel striking), this will slowly destroy the cartilage in your knees, even with padded running shoes. Furthermore, the impact pressure wave of heel striking climbs up your legs, to counteract the systolic pressure wave sending blood down your legs toward your feet.

Developing my increasingly low impact running style is one of my ongoing priorities. Probably always will be.

Low impact walking and running took me about six months to master. I did this fifteen years ago, after two running-related knee surgeries. I successfully started over, by combining Danny Dreyer's *"Chi Running"* with Jack Heggie's *"Running with the Whole Body."* Danny Dreyer has also published a book on *"Chi Walking,"* by the way.

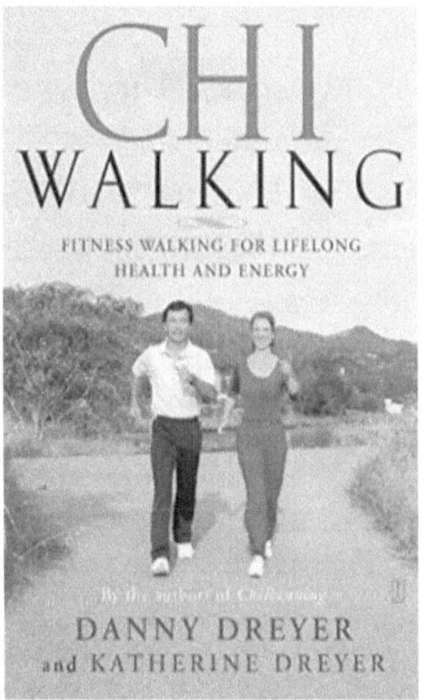

Danny Dreyer's book on Chi Running played a huge role in my ability to run injury free, after two running-related knee surgeries. I had to start over.

Important Note: If you don't trigger the discomfort

of mild claudication as you press on with your walk, your body won't know it needs to do anything, and the anything it needs to do is grow you a bunch of collaterals.

Cadence: *The total number of steps you take per minute.*

Walking and running cadence are really important. Runners talk about cadence a lot whereas I rarely hear walkers mention it. I've noticed that there are two kinds of walkers.

Slow walkers, like myself: They have a cadence of about 40 strides per minute.

Fast walkers, who leave me in the dust: About 60 strides per minute. But they still look relaxed!

Find your ideal pace, choose walking partners with a similar pace, and work to increase your cadence gradually. Make small increases from your natural cadence, little-by-little. No more than 5% per week - going from 40 to 42 or 60 to 63 strides per minute. This exercise is designed to trigger claudication or other PAD symptoms. Then your body will know it has collaterals to grow.

This is no different to any other kind of physical or sports training, which I base on the 10% rule, a well-known approach to safer run training.

***The 10-percent rule** (10PR) is one of the most important and time-proven running principles. It states that you should never increase your weekly mileage by more than 10 percent over the previous week.*

— Runner's World

I know this is working, because I have nice pink toes, even though a vascular surgery resident couldn't find a pulse in my right foot recently, even with ultrasound. My right foot seems to be running on collaterals I've built over a lifetime of physical training.

By-the-Way, *when it hurts don't complain about it.* To quote one of my Ironman coaches, Chris Hauth, *"This is training camp, not complaining camp!"*

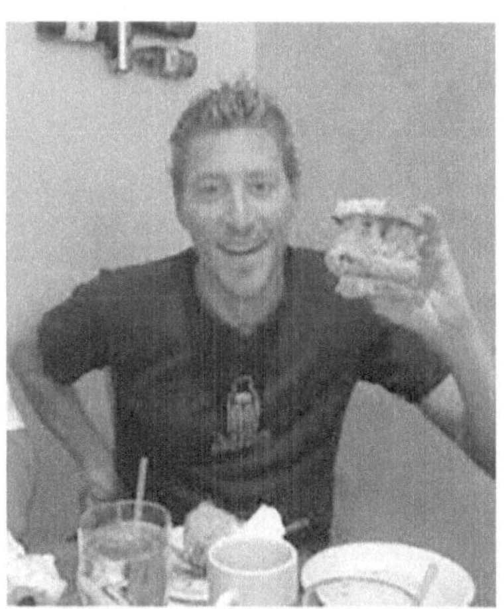

Chris is a great Ironman coach, but he does not suffer whiners gladly.

If you decide to hire a coach find one who understands PAD and knows what the hell they are talking about. Enough said!

Walk on brave soul, for your feet and your future.

I can hear some people saying, *"What if you are already on your feet all day, like a floor nurse for instance?"* They spend their day walking all over the hospital. In this case the only option is to change the way you walk, but it will most certainly be a challenge. This is a real conundrum I need to think about more.

Onto my most effective idea, one that really works.

5

STEP FIVE: FLEX YOUR TOES

Flex your toes to improve venous return.

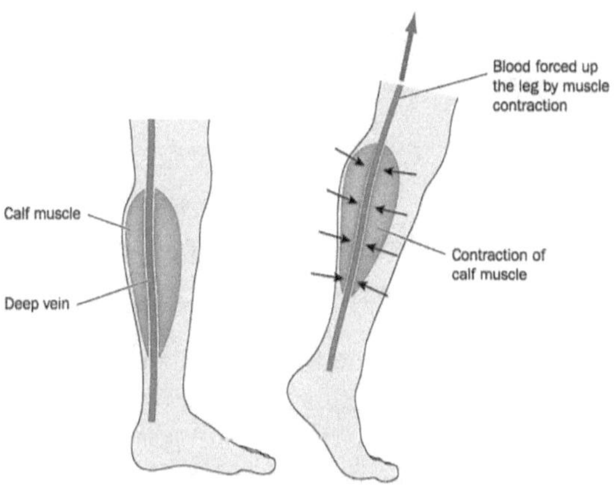

*Contraction of calf muscles squeezes veins, which
have valves that prevent back flow. This is how
muscle contraction improves venous return by
pumping blood back toward your heart.*

While running a hill a few months ago my right calf started to complain so I eased my pace back, then a thought popped into my head. I wondered if I could use muscle action to increase blood flow toward my heart as I run. To improve venous return.

I stopped running and felt my calves as I flexed my toes. Toe flexion, as in picking up a paper towel by curling your toes down around it, induced clear contraction of my calf muscles. I then noticed that I could control which muscles contracted by selecting the toes I flexed.

Flexion (medical)
A bending movement around a joint in a limb (as the knee or elbow) that decreases the angle between the bones of the limb at the joint.

— Merriam Webster Online Dictionary

The following plumbing 101 thoughts passed through my mind, as I stood there:

"Maybe I can gently flex my toes as I run, which will contract the associated muscles, and pump blood out of the veins in my calves and feet as veins have valves. This would reduce back pressure, making it easier for the flow of incoming arterial blood.

But that would compress the arteries too, which would slow blood delivery to my feet.

Wait a minute. Veins are thin walled and under low blood pressure and thus more easily compressed than arteries that are under higher internal blood pressure and have thicker walls than veins and are thus less compressible. What if I contracted my calf muscles gently enough to encourage venous return, while not contracting them hard enough to have a significant effect on the arterial blood delivery."

It's how my pathology brain works, aided by years of studying anatomy, physiology and fluid mechanics. This is how you need to start thinking once your surgeons have done all they can.

"Better do some research to see if there are any data to support this idea."

I headed home, got onto PubMed, a huge free open science database, and immediately found an encouraging article, entitled *"Effects of muscle contraction on skeletal muscle blood flow: when is there a muscle pump?"* The results were from studies in rats. What's good enough for rats is good enough for me, as we are only separated from rats evolutionarily by about 80 million years! The conclusion of the article said *"The muscle pump* [venous compression] *contributes to the initial increase in blood flow at exercise onset and to maintenance of blood flow during exercise."*

Encouraging! Then I came across this interesting blog post about humans rather than rats:

"When the calf muscle contracts, blood is squeezed out of the veins and pushed along the venous system. One-way valves in the leg veins keep the blood flowing in the correct direction toward the heart. These valves also prevent gravity from pulling blood back down your leg's veins in the wrong direction."

— blog YOUR SECOND HEART, Vein Atlanta

I soon found that gently flexing my toes as I ran allowed me to run further before calf claudication set in. It simultaneously created strain on my anterior shin muscles. This is why you have to listen to your body and make changes slowly. *I had to learn how to get the degree of toe flexion just right, while coordinating this action with my stride,* to gently squeeze those veins, while not interfering with arterial flow or straining something.

A few days later I went on a 10-mile training walk, which usually involves my having to stop for a calf blood refill on some of the hills, or to back off a lot on my pace. To my delight, as long as I kept up gentle toe flexions just as my feet encountered the ground, basically stroking the inside of my shoe with the tips of my toes, I didn't need to *"stop for gas."*

Of all the things I've learned over the last few years,

this was the most exciting. It enables me to run with few if any blood refill stops, improving my run performance and definitely improving my mood. Who wants to stop while they are out on a run, especially during a race, I'd like to know?

That said, it's a tricky business that takes practice, time and patience.

6

———

STEP SIX: STAY FLEXIBLE AND BALANCED

Hone your flexibility and balance for movement efficiency.

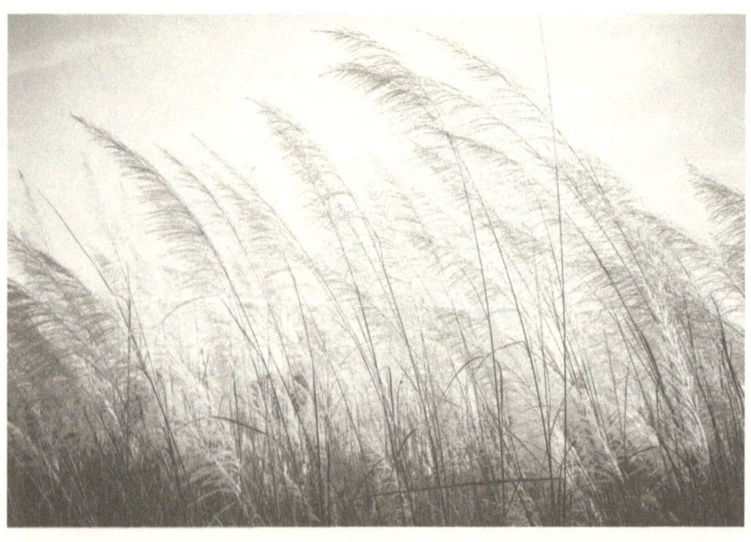

"The hard and stiff will be broken,
The soft and supple will prevail."

— *Tao Te Ching: A New English Version (Perennial Classics)*
by Stephen Mitchell

It is so important to maintain flexibility and balance as you age. Just look around at all those stiff old people, walking as if they are afraid they might fall over. I often wonder how the hell they get out of bed in the morning. Even though I'm nearly 80 years old, my approach is to work on flexibility and balance every day.

Stretching for Flexibility

The Stretch Reflex

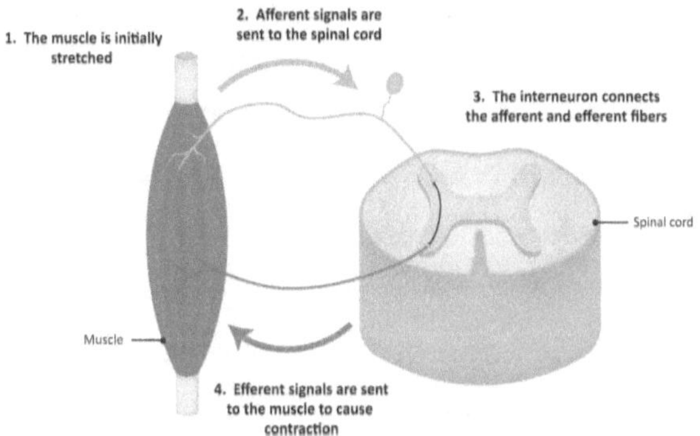

You have to be gentle to avoid triggering this spinal reflex arc.

Don't apply excessive force when stretching muscles to lengthen or relax them. This has to be done gently. There are several ways to effectively increase muscle length and thus your flexibility. A better term for "stretching" is "lengthening." If you pull sharply on a muscle it will reflexly contract to protect itself from tearing. This is achieved through the spinal circuitry shown above.

It's also important to warm up your muscles before you stretch them.

To get started sit on the floor and without straining your lower back try touching your toes. You'll immediately see how much work you have to do on your hamstrings and hips. Furthermore, we get tighter as we age. This is why I stretch after every workout, when standing in line (I do get funny looks), while waiting to cross the road (my little dog ignores me), or any time I get a chance.

Remember:

"Stretching is a conversation you have with your body, not something you do to your body."

Stretching is not a duty, a job, a pain in the ass, an unpleasant thing you do to yourself. Stretching is an interesting chat with your best friend, your body.

There are many places to learn about the art of stretching. You could start with a Yoga class or explore Active Isolated Stretching, both of which are highly effective approaches to maintaining your flexibility.

Whatever you do stretch gently. You can over-stretch and injure yourself while stretching. However, if you don't build stretching into your daily routine you'll pull a tight muscle, eventually.

Damned if you do, damned if you don't?

That thought made me laugh and laughter really is the best medicine. Don't do it while stretching or you might yank something!

I'm still laughing!

Most of my stretching sessions last five to 20 minutes. I occasionally undertake one-hour stretching sessions when in full training. Stretch to gently lengthen those muscles, loosen joints, tone connective tissue, wake up your mind, *and don't forget to stay well hydrated.* If you can afford it, a sports massage will find your tight muscles, it will tell you which muscles need a little chat. Where you need to do some muscle lengthening.

Now for another oft-neglected issue that really does impact our old age and our fight against PAD.

Balance

For balance as you age adequate hydration is extremely important.

I hope you will excuse my quoting myself. I lifted the following section from one of my previous books,

"How to Train for Aging: The Ultimate Endurance Sport." It's not too bad so why reinvent the wheel?

BALANCE WELL TO WALK WELL, *run well, swim well, and generally get around well.*

I practice balance daily and I don't let blinding light impair my balance work, as is explained below.

Vision makes us blind

Each morning in the winter I awake to a nice warm cat on my feet, a dog huddled up to my side, and a wood stove needing attention. What's new? Gizmo, Cat and I would freeze pretty quickly in our tiny house without this little wood stove. I go outside, one step away, to a world that is quiet and dark with Orion's belt overhead telling me the time. I step back into the growing warmth of our cosy little house, stand at the window and do my routine balance exercise.

Standing, feet together, eyes closed.

Listening! I hear them talking to me. Those amazing balance sensors: somatic, inner ear, soles of my feet.

- *Somatic – Pressure on muscles, tendons, ligaments and joints, as my body sways around that straight line of gravity extending from outer space, through my body to the center of the*

Earth. I guess it's not really straight, but I'll have to think about that in terms of all that Einstein relativity stuff. Let's assume it is straight because it feels straight as a plumb line and those somatic sensors tell me if I'm falling off that line.

- ***Inner ear** – The magic machinery of my semicircular canals tells me I'm upright and moving around gently as my feet and ankles correct my center of gravity with barely detectable muscle contractions and relaxations around my ankles.*

- ***Soles of my feet** – Thousands of mechanoreceptors detect local pressure, vibration and shear, to tell my brain, maybe not even my brain, perhaps only local nerve pathways that pass through my spinal cord, how to fine tune my position in space. Sensors send signals through nerves to my spinal cord which, like a policeman directing traffic, then sends messages thorough other nerves to muscles in my lower legs, telling them how to adjust their local tension to refine my balance, all based on messages from the soles of my feet.*

Then I open my eyes to see the stars and I'm suddenly blind elsewhere. My other senses of balance are over-whelmed by my powerful sense of vision. My mind automatically selects a light across the way and locks in like a laser-

guided missile. I immediately sway less and my stance is more solid, less fluid, less of a physical dance. My body becomes more rigid.

Our powerful sense of vision blinds us to our other three balance systems. Learning how to tune into all four by practicing with our eyes closed is essential for physical stability as we age. You might be stumbling around in the dark one night and take a fall because you neglected to train your non-vision-related balance machinery.

A final note on balance: As I age I've noticed that maintaining hydration is increasingly critical. That became apparent as I headed for the shore for a recent race and nearly fell as I toppled to my right. It was a cold day and still dark. A day when one doesn't think to drink enough water. I took a quick gulp from my water bottle, fixed my eyes on dimly lit stable objects around me, and continued cautiously toward the swim start, and stability quickly returned because of my intake of water. One fall can ruin your day so beware.

On balance, as I age, I think balance is one of my most valuable assets, even more than flexibility and loving to learn new stuff. Lose your balance and your life falls apart. You can't even read, what a terrible thought.

A Note on Tension - It Spreads

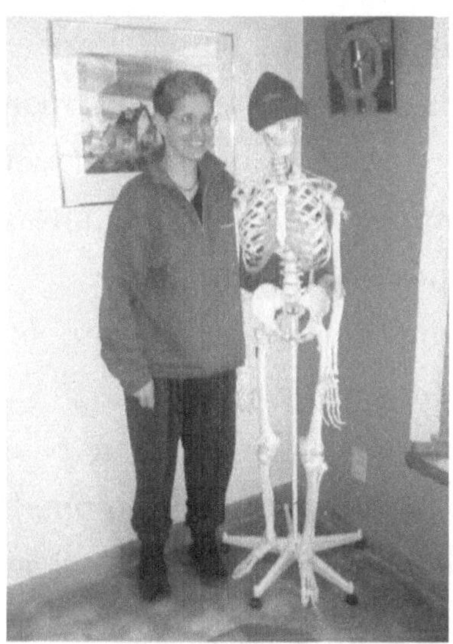

Karen and her assistant, Mr. Bones

I studied Feldenkrais for many years with a wonderful teacher, Karen, and her assistant Mr. Bones. This training transformed my body movement, flexibility and balance.

The Feldenkrais Method® of somatic education uses gentle movement and directed attention to help people learn new and more effective ways of living the life they want. You can increase your ease and range of motion, improve your flexibility and coordination, and rediscover your innate capacity for graceful, efficient movement.

— Feldenkrais Method, at feldenkrais.com

Occasionally I would join a group class. In one such class, there were about ten adults of all ages, men and women. A friendly, happy bunch. Karen asked us all to walk around near the center of the room however we wanted. Everyone smiled and relaxed, while wondering what was coming next. There was always some weird thing coming next in Feldenkrais.

Then Karen said *"Now tense your right fist. Tense it as tight as you can and continue walking."*

At first nothing changed, then people started to stumble. One person bumped into me. He apologized. All of us started to walk in a much stiffer way, having to concentrate on not running into others.

After a few minutes of increasingly weird walking, Karen said, *"Now relax that hand."*

Before we knew it we were walking around normally and easily again.

Karen said, *"Now you can see how tension spreads. Both physical and mental tension."*

Don't let tension become a friend of your PAD. Pain-induced tension is literally your enemy when it comes to enjoying a walk or a run.

Tension is not your friend.

When claudication pain strikes, fight to relax that tight muscle. You are fighting a reflex designed to protect a muscle in pain due to loss of blood supply, but this muscle tension only makes things worse. You can fight this unhelpful reflex with a strong mind and strong muscles.

This is why strength training is an important part of PAD training.

Core Strength Is Critical For Balance

Your core is a region of your body around your pelvis, the strength and health of which is extremely impor-tant for your stability and mobility. There are many core exercises well worth your time exploring, as it's too big a topic to cover in this book. I do show my favorite daily core exercise in the FitOldDog Video Channel, under the title *"BODY MOVEMENT FOR AGING: The Art Of Stretching For Flexibility As You Age."*

Here is an excellent description of your core

The core is the part of the human body located between the pelvic floor and diaphragm, and its main job is to hold and protect your spine. Your abdominal muscles are part of your core, but just one piece of the puzzle. The core muscles squeeze, or hug, the spine, almost like a hand would squeeze a tube of toothpaste, taking pressure off the body. These muscles, and there are many of them in this area of your musculature, work hard together to achieve balance in your spine.

Besides being a primary stabilizer of the body, another reason the core muscles are different from other muscles is because they move across three planes of motion. Rather than being restricted to only moving in certain directions, they work together as a three-dimensional whole to support and stabilize you as you pile them with work every day. They anticipate and react to stress on the body and are able to work together to balance the load.

See why a strong core is so important?

— Ortho Carolina, *Why the Core Muscles are Different from Other Muscles*

THE MUSCLES of your core include the *transverse abdominis, multifidus,* internal and external obliques, *erector spinae,* muscles of the diaphragm and pelvic floor, *rectus abdominis (six pack muscles), latissimus dorsi, trapezius,* and your glutes (butt muscles). I said it's complicated, but you don't need to memorize them, you have to get to know and feel them. I exercise my core regularly, and I use a simple balance test to check their fitness.

When my core is strong the exercise below has little or no impact on my balance. If my core is weak I fall all over the place because I can't stabilize my spine and hips. Work to do!

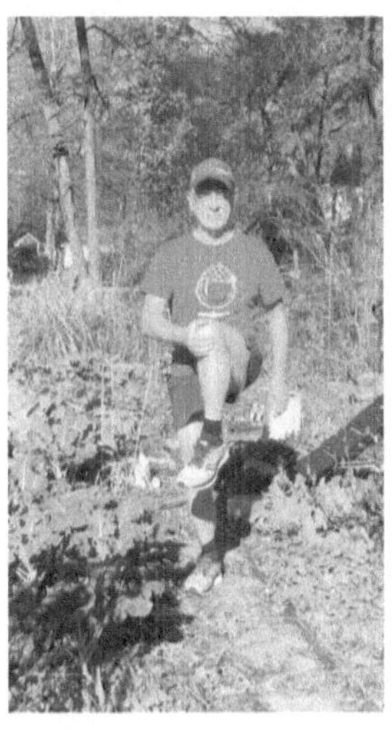

I lock my pelvis by pulling my knee toward my midline,
as a balance test of my core strength.

This is a life-long study in itself but some simple exercises can dramatically improve core strength. If your core is weak when you stand on one leg your hips will flail around and you'll lose your balance. When your core is strong your pelvis remains stable, and you can balance easily on one leg with your eyes open. *With practice with your eyes closed.*

If pulling my knee toward my center line, to lock my pelvis, as in the image above, markedly improves my balance, I have core work to do.

7

STEP SEVEN: INCREASE YOUR STRENGTH

"Underneath tightness, lies weakness."

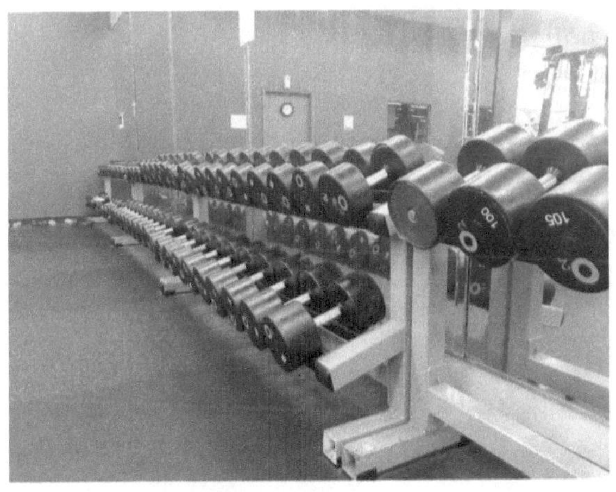

I can only give you a taste of the subject of strength training for PAD but I can convey my training philosophy. I already covered core which you should visit at least briefly almost every time you use the weight room. Don't be overwhelmed. I didn't know squat about squats when I started strength training in a weight room 50 years ago.

Oops! It was 60 years ago. Damn! I'm old!

Patiently learn new skills and fight the monster, PAD, with your mind, body and spirit. Your body is on your side, believe it or not, while your mind might take a while to get with the program. I address spirit in chapter twelve. It's in the nature of our ego to fight change due to its obsession with security and safety, thus one of my favorite words:

Misoneism

Fear of change.

If you wish to overcome lower limb PAD and kill the monster you'll have to get your whole body in on the act, while putting out some effort. There are several aspects to strength conditioning. I'll address each briefly as this will become one of your life-long weapons against pain and dysfunction. Don't worry! You'll find a way to make it fun. I love going to the weight room, where I feel quite at home. It just takes time. It's best if they are hot, noisy and busy.

Your Mind

The first thing I do before strength training is warm up on an elliptical trainer. No rowing machine allowed with an AAA as it could displace my stent. Bummer!

Before you start turn off the damn TV and take out those earbuds.

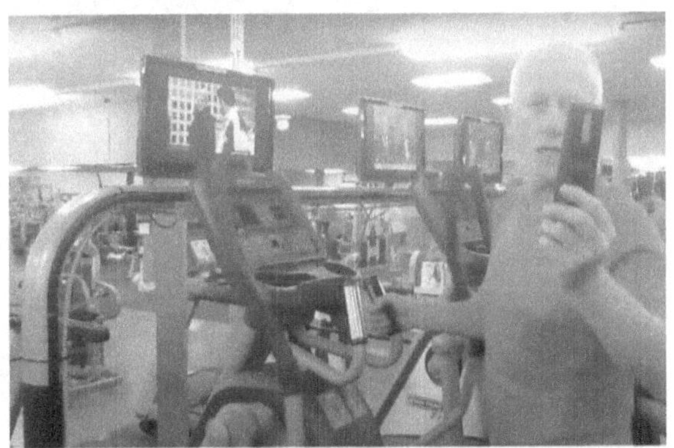

Training requires focus.

You will need to develop the necessary habits.

The only way to train your mind to condition your body is through routine, through slowly built habits. I do this in the swimming pool, on the bike, running on the road, and working in the weight room. Consistently!

"Dream, then do!" is my mantra.

Did you know that thinking about exercising can make you fitter? Sorry! With PAD you need to do more than think. Find a weight room, go with a friend or alone, and read some books on weight training (not weight lifting). Get with the program and your mind will step up to the plate. You might consider reading this inspiring book if you doubt your ability to change your mind.

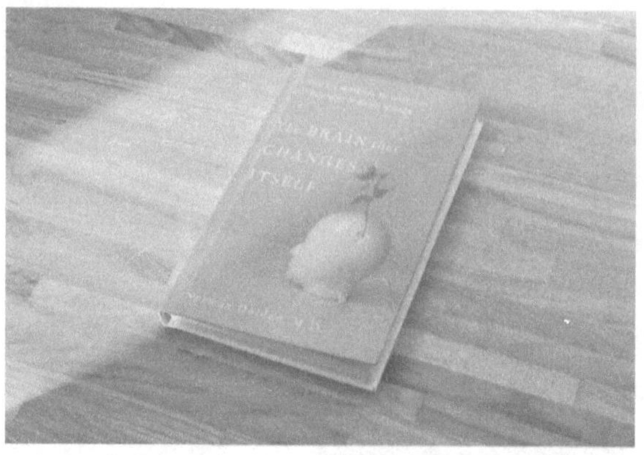

"The Mind That Changes Itself" *will encourage you to learn new things to fight PAD.*

Those 100-mile bike rides sure train my mental conditioning.

Your Cardiovascular System

With your newly conditioned mind it's time to start *cardio* (heart) *vascular* (arteries, arterioles, capillaries, venules, veins, lymphatics, and probably stuff I forgot) *conditioning.* This requires pushing yourself little by little, as you need to get your heart rate up. Certain drugs can prevent you from doing this. Whether you choose to condition your cardiovascular system or take those drugs is up to you.

I consider training, diet, mental attitude and kindness to myself and others, to be my most important medications.

How much and how fast you increase your heart rate depends on your health and your goals. Some may need medical supervision. I make modest increases in my heart rate and perceived effort during cardio training. No more than 5-10% increase in load per week. I do this mainly in the pool and on the bike. For running my cardio training is confined to hill repeats on short hills with a moderate incline of no more than 3% grade. I then walk back down to let blood refill my calves and feet. Then I do it again until I've had enough, which is a judgement call based on my training level at the time. You may consider hiring a trained coach familiar with the challenges of PAD. I've never met such a coach, by the way.

Important note:

Don't think of the cardiovascular system as a single pump, the heart, and a bunch of pipes the heart forces blood through. Nothing could be further from the truth. It is a highly integrated system of many pumps. For starters, the human heart consists of two pumps, the left and right side. The former sends blood to the

body, the latter to the lungs, though it is more complicated than that. Everything is, when you delve deeper.

Many pumps?

Yes, thousands of pumps!

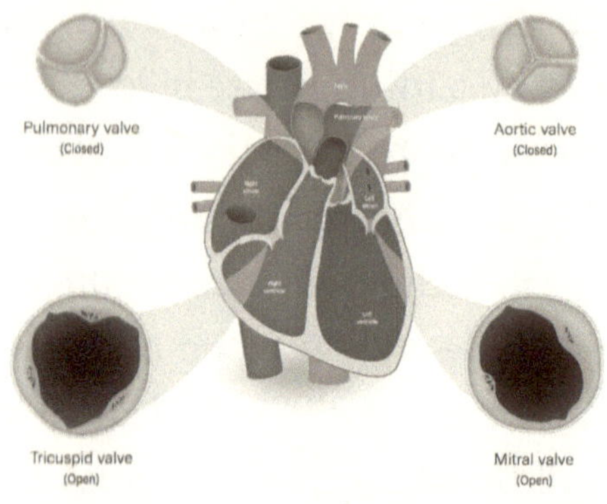

The heart during diastole (relaxing) to show how the
aortic arch is yet another pump (see below).

I already mentioned in Chapter 5 how muscle
contraction in my calves, induced by flexing my toes,
improves venous return as I run. This is because veins
have valves, which permits this pumping action.

When the strong left ventricle contracts (systole), it
sends blood into the highly elastic aortic arch. This
contraction squeezes most of the blood out of the heart
muscle. Then the left ventricle relaxes, the aortic valve
slams shut, and the aortic arch is now loaded with
blood under pressure, which pumps blood into the

heart muscle. The heart can hardly pump blood into itself, while contracting.

As the muscles of the ventricles relax (diastole), their muscles are more easily perfused with blood. The stored pressure in the aortic arch pumps its blood into the relaxing heart muscle and to the rest of the body. The aortic arch is yet another pump.

Did you know: *Exercise encourages the growth of new blood vessels, collaterals, in your heart, helping to keep heart disease at bay. Chances are if you have PAD you should keep an eye on your heart health, too.*

The entire 100,000 miles of arteries, capillaries, and veins in your body, act as pumps, one way or another. You might ask about those microscopic capillaries that provide blood to the tissues. They use osmotic pumps. We have muscle contraction, elastic storage, and osmosis, all acting as pumps in your cardiovascular system. It's one magical machine, a plumbing machine, and one you should study as you fight PAD. A little education goes a long way.

Body movement is critical for our survival as we age. Become physically weak, fall over, break a hip, and die in bed. Screw that, I say!

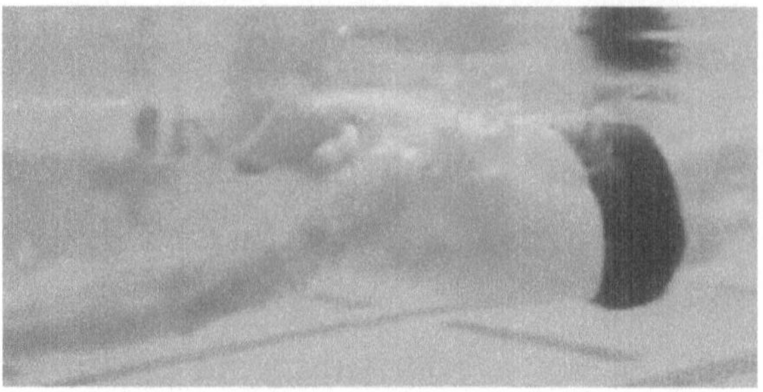

I've been swimming for over 70 years!

I find my best cardiovascular training is done in the pool. I can hammer out laps with no calf or foot pain, to get my heart rate up. If you are not a swimmer I suggest you consider water running, with or without a float aid, which is demonstrated in my YouTube channel, under the title *"Water Running by FitOldDog."*

I suggest you start with a float aid, then slowly dump it as your skill improves. You can use your open hands to keep you up at first, but after a while that becomes unnecessary.

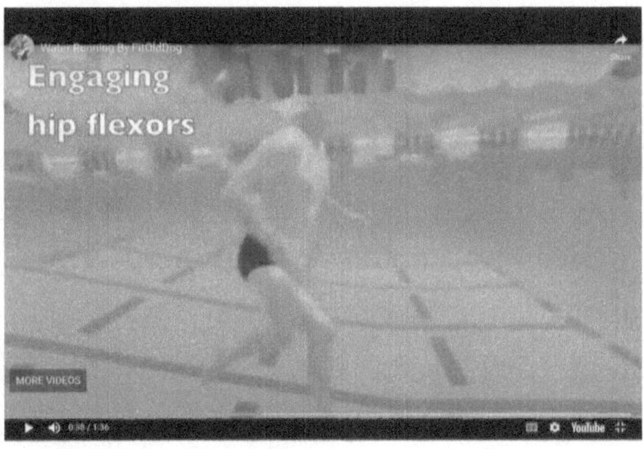

*Yours truly water running. It is tougher than it looks,
especially without a float aid.*

Your Muscles And Other Connective Tissues

You are made up of a bunch of connective tissues, which form an integrated physical machine, you. These tissues include muscles, bones, nerves, ligaments, tendons, lymphatics, and so on, and they are alive. Even your bones are alive. They most certainly are alive, and you don't want to go thinking otherwise. Treat them with the respect they deserve, and they'll serve you well.

It's unwise to think about the bits of your body like bits of a car. Car bits aren't alive, they can't fix themselves. You can build new blood vessels, those magical collaterals, because your blood vessels are alive.

As you start working out in the gym, which is a good idea, doing weight training (not weight lifting), calisthenics, push ups, pull ups, whatever, you are toughening all of your connective tissues, not just muscles, but bones, cartilage, tendons, ligaments, and so on, as well. You have to pace yourself, and never use steroids to accelerate muscle growth, which will outpace growth of ligaments and tendons. I've heard some horror stories about steroid use in my local gym.

Explore how your body responds to load and toughen it up, slowly and patiently. I've been working in weight rooms for over 60 years, and I still learn new tricks. I learned one the other day, when I noticed a woman doing *one arm bent rows with a 20lb. dumbbell, from high plank, supported on the other arm.* That is a tough core workout, I tried it. You will slowly learn the lingo, don't worry.

Most importantly: If you have a stent as I do in my aorta, make sure your workouts don't put it at risk. This was important for me as I resumed Ironman training with an AAA stent graft. I had to abandon the rowing machine for warmups and minimize hip flexion on the bike, for instance.

Many people are shy and disoriented when they first use a weight room. Don't give a damn about people watching you. They are only thinking about themselves anyway.

Free weights are far superior to machines for weight training, in my opinion.

I've not idea which exercises will work best for you, as we are all different. For instance, I used to lift weights with my three sons. When it came to bench press, two were comfortable with the bar, while in the case of my third son the bar gave him severe shoulder pain. So he used dumbbells. Dumbbells don't lock the movement into one path through the shoulder joint.

This is also true for the bike, which is why I like pedals with plenty of "float." Even made a crude video about it on YouTube, entitled *"SpeedPlay Pedals Can Help Your Knees on the Bike.* I made it with my old Blackberry and it has over 16,000 views, already.

One guy complained that I had hairy legs. I'm a guy, what did he expect? You can't satisfy some people, in fact if you satisfy everyone you probably aren't doing anything useful.

Thus one of my favorite quotes:

'The reasonable man adapts himself to the world; the unreasonable man persists in trying to adapt the world to himself. Therefore all progress depends on the unreasonable man.'

— George Bernard Shaw

One final example: strengthening your pesky hamstrings.

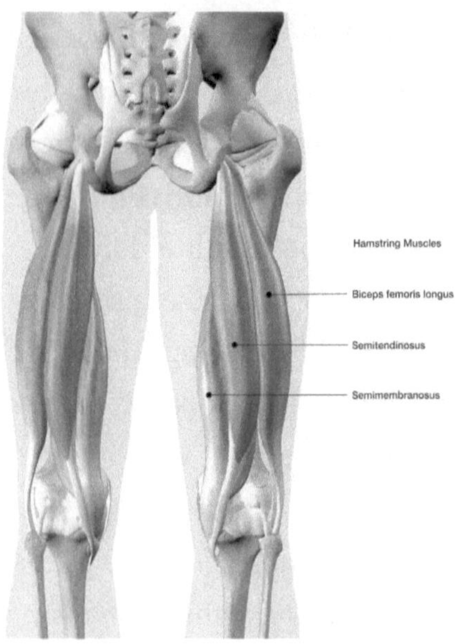

The hamstring muscles.

I know at least six hamstring exercises, but I prefer deadlifts. They work better than the other exercises I've tried, especially the machines that feel as though they might break my hamstrings. Make sure to learn the anatomy of each muscle you are trying to improve, and don't forget to stretch after each workout, please. Yank a hamstring and you'll be in trouble, because you failed to show respect.

Enjoy getting stronger every day!

8

———

STEP EIGHT: PICK UP YOUR PACE

Increase pace to induce claudication and grow those foot saving collaterals.

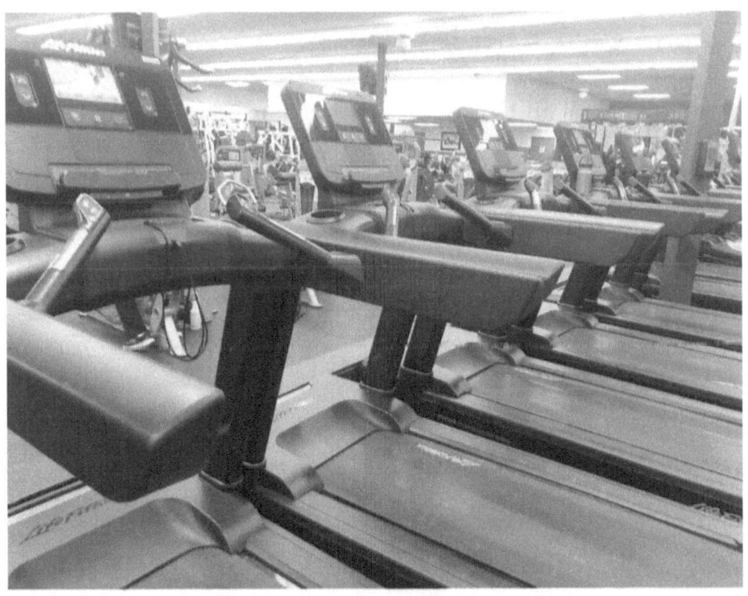

Indoor treadmills are invaluable for PAD training during inclement weather. They are also useful for improving your walking pace before doing so on the unforgiving roads and trails. Treadmill walking and running is easier on your body, and it is ideal for working on your whole-body walking skills.

Whenever I try a modification to my run, to improve blood flow through my calves and feet, I start on a treadmill before migrating to the road. Right now, I'm working on a treadmill to eliminate one remaining corn on my right foot, the one by my little toe. Developing optimal foot mechanics with a limited blood supply is tricky, but I'm getting there.

There is no way I can fully compensate for blocked popliteal arteries. Collaterals go a long way toward supplying much needed blood to my lower legs, but it's never quite the same, thus the need for optimal mechanics.

You can find treadmills all over the place, so go find one, Do some work and have fun too! When you are ready start to pick up your cadence on the treadmill and then while walking outside. You have to focus. As you increase pace the skills you recently mastered, such as soft spread feet, can fall apart as claudication rears its ugly head. This is why it's important to increase cadence gradually. Take yourself to the edge of dysfunction, while still being able to walk or run.

9

STEP NINE: EAT RIGHT

You are what you eat when it comes to PAD.

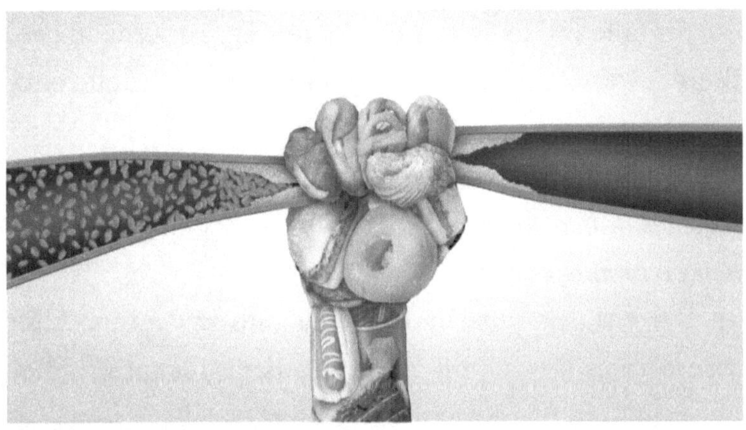

D iet can contribute to the development of blocked arteries due to fat buildup, or it can make a genetic tendency, as in my case, worse. Fortunately, I've been vegetarian for years, but prior to that I ate whatever I liked, from fatty dairy products to fatty steaks. Maybe that contributed to where I am today.

As we tend to develop PAD later in life, many of us have other issues going on. I've generally been lucky health wise, in part due to persistent exercise and more recently to a vegetarian diet. I started a strict vegan diet six years ago. Within weeks of going off of dairy products my prostate hyperplasia symptoms vanished, never to return, so far. Everything was fine until after three years on the vegan diet I developed terrible nose bleeds (epistaxis). Blood would flood out of my right nostril at the most inconvenient times. An Ear, Nose and Throat doctor failed to fix it, so I tried a few eggs a week in case there was an underlying nutritional deficiency going on.

My Mum used to say, *"Those doctors are wrong about eggs being bad for us. Eggs contain everything needed to make a complete chick."*

I think this put the egg idea into my mind. After several eggs a week my nose bleeds disappeared, They have yet to return several years later.

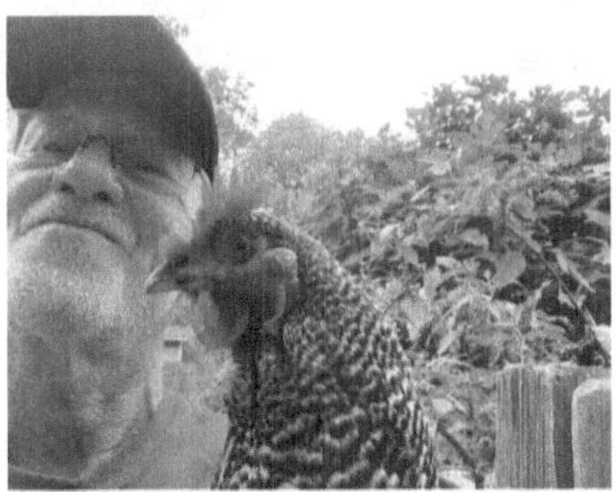

*Thanks for saving me from that terrible epistaxis,
Galaxy.*

If diet eliminated my prostate hyperplasia symptoms, then both induced and cured my nose bleeds, can diet impact PAD symptoms? You bet! Logic would suggest that diet could be an important issue when it comes to PAD. Fortunately, Kym McNicholas recently published a whole book on the topic, *"Food For Thought."*

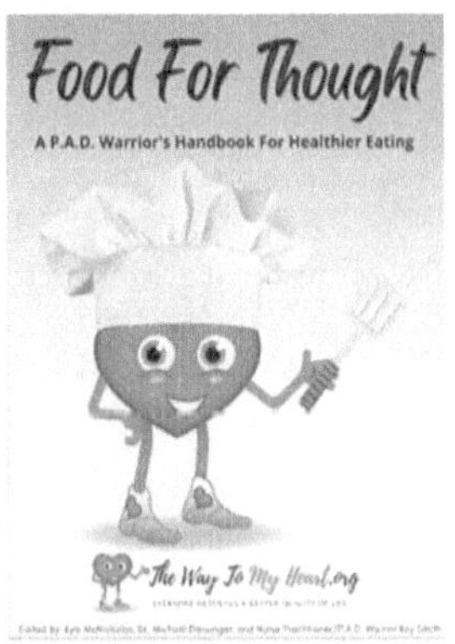

My recommendation is that you eat as healthily as you are able. When it comes to diet, your body knows best, but you have to get beyond old habits and conditioning, and quiet your mind to hear what your body is telling you.

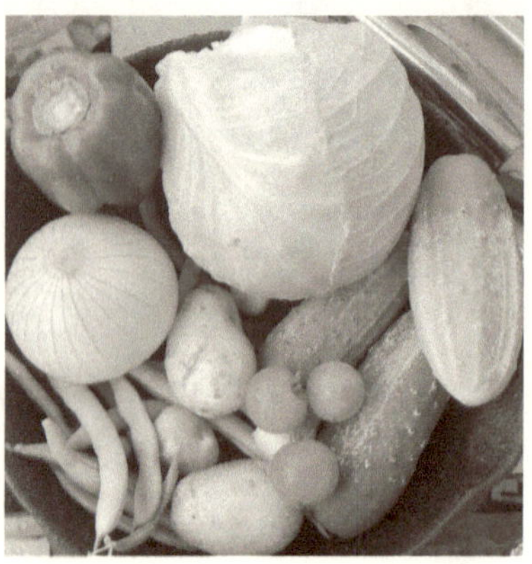

Some fresh veg from my garden.

A vegetable garden is another way to fight PAD, which I supplement with eggs from these lovely ladies.

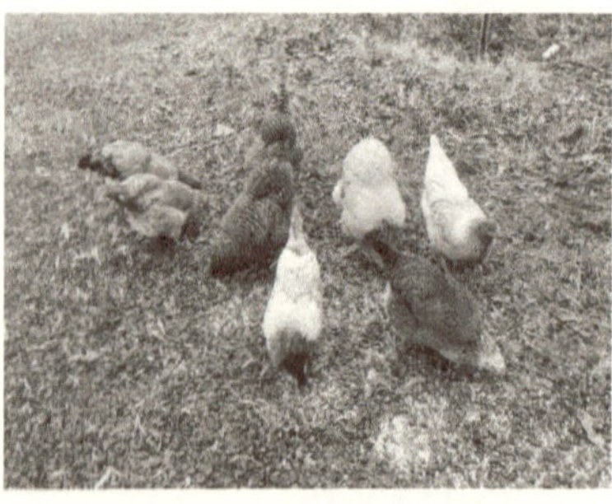

Galaxy, Dipa, Denali, Falconer, Citra, Chinook, Jade, and Bertha, thanks so much for fixing my epistaxis.

I've no intention of eating those chickens when they

stop laying, unless there's an apocalypse. They are my friends.

Bon appétit!

10

STEP TEN: MASTER NOT THINKING

True skill leads to not thinking.

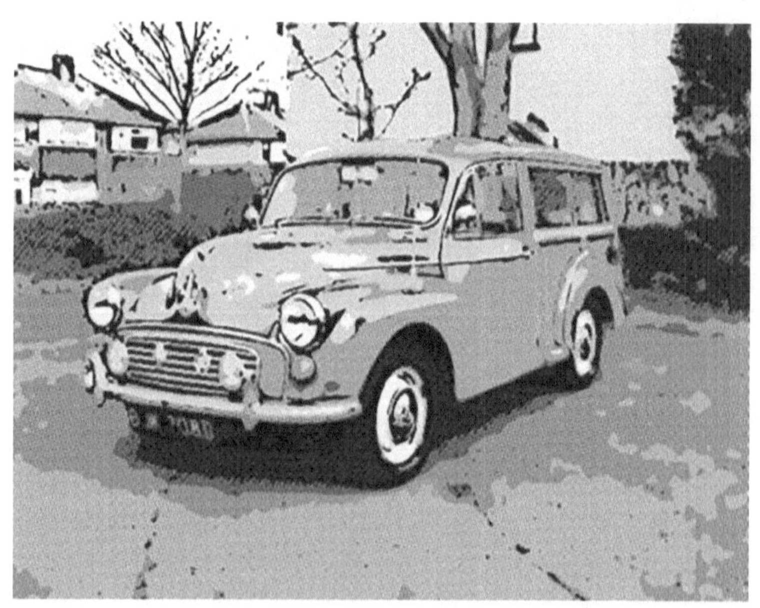

My first car as a young veterinarian in England, back in 1967.

Do you remember learning how to drive? If you don't drive think of something else you learned that was challenging, like playing a musical instrument (for me the flute) or a foreign language (I still enjoy reading French literature). I spent years "mastering" the flute and French, but driving was another matter. I had a crash course.

After four years as a student I qualified as a veterinarian in 1967, in Bristol, England. At that time I only drove a motorbike. It never occurred to me to learn to drive a car. I had six weeks from graduation before starting work in a local veterinary practice, a job I accepted without a thought about driving. I don't think it was even mentioned in my interview.

I had to pass the driving test before I could work on farms scattered around the City of Bristol and throughout the Cotswold Hills. I could only afford a few lessons, but I passed the test anyway. No idea how I did that. The British driving test was really challenging back then.

When driving I had to think about everything I did. Steering, maintaining speed while avoiding other drivers, braking in time. These were all conscious decisions as a neophyte driver. That first week I drove over 500 miles from farm to farm, from sick dog to sick cat to sick guinea pig. I knew how to drive, but it wasn't running on autopilot in my subconscious. This left me completely exhausted along with some close calls on the road.

At the end of that first week I was more exhausted, mentally, than I had ever been in my life. I had to think about everything I did, as a neophyte vet and inexperienced car driver.

You may wonder why I'm talking about this. Because we are at step 10, and you will need to load steps 1-9 into your subconscious through dedicated repetition. That's what I did, anyway, and it seems to be working.

The work described in this book involves multiple steps. Each one is relatively easy to learn and to do, *on its own*. Like turning the steering wheel in your car, while putting pressure on the brake pedal, and checking your wing mirrors, plus sipping a coffee. No big deal, right? Now you are learning to drive your body, which has a steering wheel and brakes, too. It took me seven years to develop and then make a subconscious habit of each of the first nine steps in this book. I had to load them into my subconscious, so I can walk and run without thinking about them.

I can't be thinking about my feet the whole time I'm walking with a friend or running a marathon.

This reminds me of a fantastic bike ride I did years ago with my triathlon coach, Chris, and fifteen other athletes. We rode from San Francisco to San Diego, along highway one with some detours, a distance of six hundred miles in five days. We were on bicycles and it only stopped raining for two hours the whole time. That's what I call training. I bet I built some collaterals during those harsh training rides.

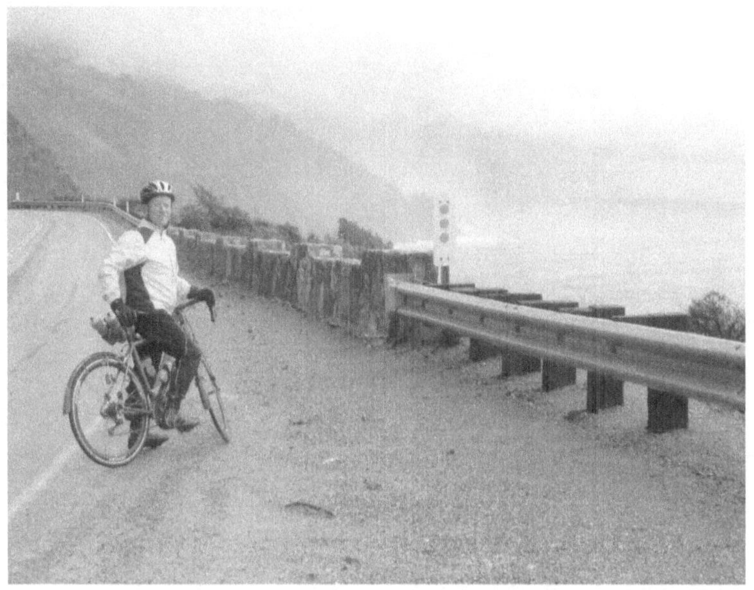

A beautiful day on Highway One, overlooking the Pacific Ocean.

We were riding in a pack, 120 miles a day, in heavy rain. One day I was admiring the view, when I chanced to glance down at my feet. The pedals were spinning as if they belonged to someone else. It was as though they weren't part of me. They were just doing their thing. I'd spun those pedals so many times I didn't need to think about it anymore.

You may ask, *"Do I have to get all the steps in this book incorporated into my subconscious?"*

Answer: *"It's probably a good idea, at least for the ones that work for you."*

It's just like learning to drive.

STEP ELEVEN: MONITOR YOUR PROGRESS

Assess your progress for direction and encouragement.

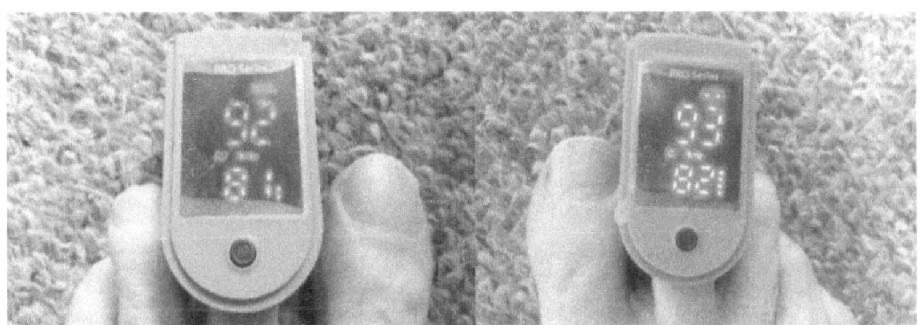

Thanks to COVID-19, I had previously purchased a $30 pulse oximeter, designed for the fingers. Seems to work well on my toes, too!

There are several ways to measure your PAD status. The surest is an ABI test as described in the *Introduction*. But this requires going to a vascular laboratory. You can assess your progress between doctor visits using the following at-home approaches.

- Foot color especially toenails.
- Blood refill rate after applying, then removing, local pressure on a toenail.
- Severity of PAD symptoms, such as claudication and foot numbness.
- Foot mechanics: are they conversing with or fighting the ground (clomp, slap, clomp)?
- Pulse oximetry: measures blood oxygen saturation level.

I published this on my blog and a fellow PAD sufferer told me his toe O2sats on his good leg was 97%, while on the problem leg it was only 80%. I recommended he head for his vascular physicians.

Being able to monitor your progress is helpful in the extreme.

STEP TWELVE: BUILD A SUPPORT TEAM

"Never give up on your dreams, no matter how painful and difficult your journey is."

— *Lalisa Manobal*, Thai rapper

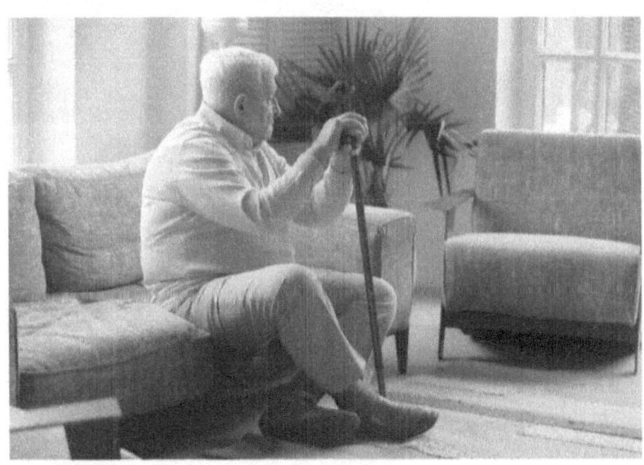

Get up! Fix that body. Dump that stick. And live, for God's sake.

We all have good days and bad days, especially with PAD. By now you may be a little overwhelmed by your pain, and by all the things I am suggesting you consider doing about it. The problem is that PAD never gives up unless it can be corrected surgically.

I'd have been dead long ago, but for that wonderful AAA stent graft from Cook Medical and the surgeons who installed it.

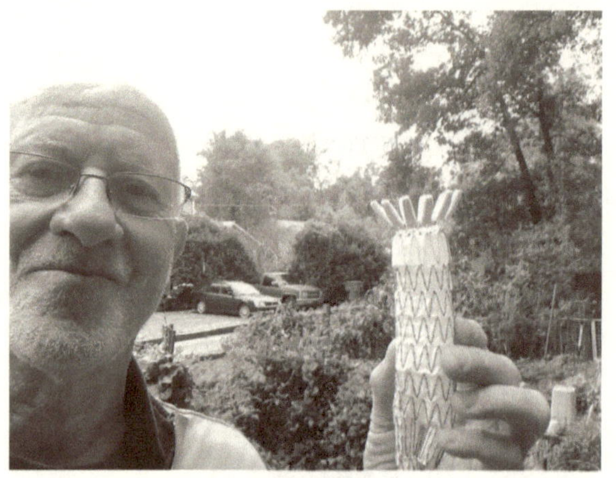

Here I am with a copy of the type of AAA stent graft I've had in my aorta since 2010. Amazing!

I kept on competing in Ironman races with that stent, and I'll be damned if I'll let PAD steal away my toes and feet. This book lays out my battle plan, but no man is an island. I have support in the form of family, friends, surgeons, vascular researchers and device manufacturers.

There is no need to go it alone if you can build a support crew. I know it isn't easy for some, but it is critical. You have to reach out.

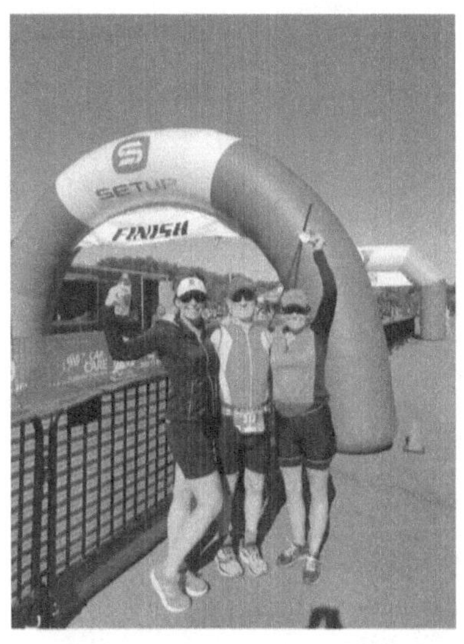

My training buddies and support crew, Maya and Tracey, after we finished a local race.

Numb feet? What the hell? Let's fix it!

Claudication? What the hell? Let's fix it!

Depressed, giving up? What the hell? Let's fix it!

How they carry out these remarkable life-saving Endovascular Aortic Repairs (EVAR) is hard to believe. You can watch how my type of AAA stent graft was inserted on YouTube, if you look around. Then Cook Medical sponsored a video team to tell the world my AAA story. It's available on YouTube under the title *"The Creation of FitOldDog."*

As Fit as I was in 2010, and in 2011 when I completed the Lake Placid Ironman with an AAA stent graft, fate was saying, *"You haven't seen anything yet, Kevin. Just wait and see what you think of PAD."*

Screw you, PAD. That's what I think of you.

AFTERWORD

Fate is like a strange, unpopular restaurant filled with odd little waiters who bring you things you never asked for and don't always like.

– Lemony Snicket

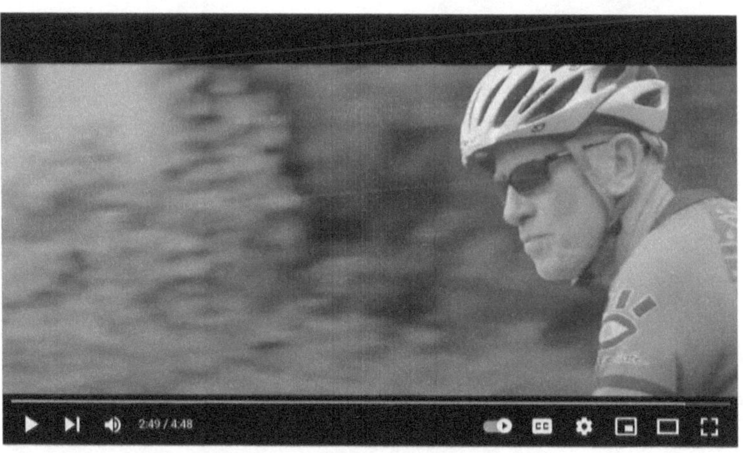

I brought all that training into my battle with PAD.

As I approach the age of 80 and look back I see that I've been fortunate to enjoy a remarkably interesting life. This came about because of my inherent curiosity. It's that gift that drives me along. It was the driving force behind the work I did for this little book, and I sure hope it helps some people out there. I've come a long way from that shy kid looking at pond water through his tiny monocular microscope back in 1946.

*I was trying to science the sh*t out of the meaning of life. Still am!*

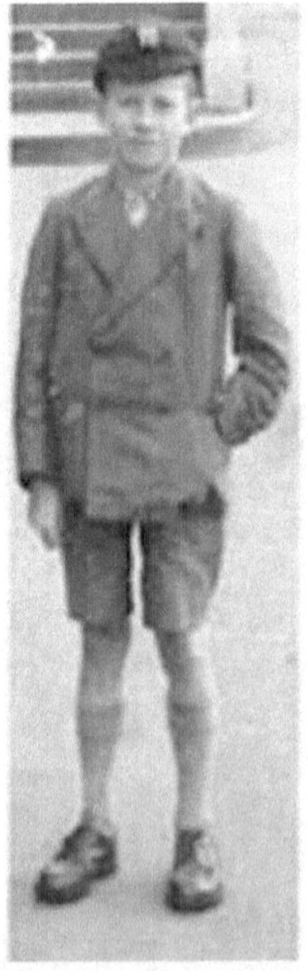 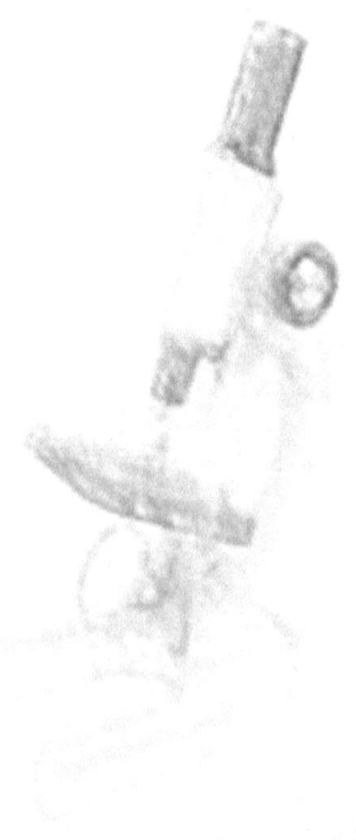

Go find inspiration and support wherever and whenever you can, and fight PAD for all your life is worth.

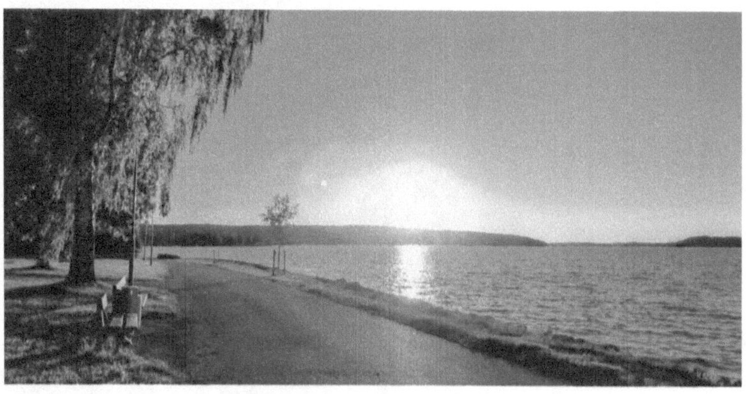

Here I come, Lahti Finland, for the August 2023 World Half Ironman Championships.

-kev

ACKNOWLEDGMENTS

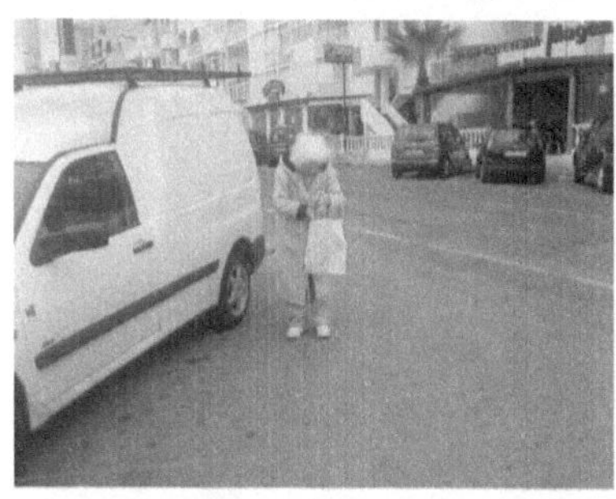

My Mum remained physically independent into her mid-90s. She taught us the importance of doing the work.

I achieved plenty, but I didn't do it alone. It truly takes a village to raise a scientist and an athlete. I have so much to be grateful for, and so many people to be grateful too, and what I am is extremely grateful. I do attempt to turn setbacks into stepping stones, because I came with the mental strength instilled into us by our mother, Joan, a real fighter. She overcame considerable odds to raise us kids as bombs were dropping and Nazi fighter jets were strafing the streets. It's funny how we rarely appreciate our parents until we face the challenges of parenting, ourselves. It's just the way of things.

Thanks, Mum!

I also want to thank my sister, Marian the Language Major, for her detailed edits. I never could master the subtle art of the comma. Thanks to Tracey for all her support at the Wilmington Half, and for agreeing to feature on the cover. I also received helpful assistance with the cover, with respect to font selection and letter spacing, from Hayley and Libby, as I am completely "font blind."

ALSO BY KEVIN THOMAS MORGAN

Self Help Aging Training Two:

A Life in Balance

Self Help

Aging Training One:

Wake Up Your Toes

Passion versus Reason On The Spectrum: An Aspergers Memoir

- Not Just Talk: Fighting Climate Change One Tiny House and Victory Garden at a Time

- Scientist in the Dark, a Novel

- We Can't Eat Grass

- How to Train for Aging: The Ultimate Endurance Sport

- The True Story of Plantar Fasciitis

- Plantar Fasciitis Has The Wrong Name

- Find Peace of Mind in the Pool

- Pain, Good Friend, Bad Master

AUTHOR'S NEWSLETTER

Old Dogs in Training LLC weekly newsletter is concerned with animal and environmental protection, fighting climate change, preparing for aging, living with vascular disease, and other subjects as they pop randomly into my head. I do have a thing for logic and lexical semantics, btw.

You can sign up for the newsletter, if you so desire, via a link at, Inspirational Self Help Books (.com), where you will also find further information on the authors publications.

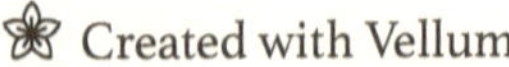 Created with Vellum

ABOUT THE AUTHOR

Kevin Thomas Morgan is a retired veterinary pathologist and research scientist. He now works on ways to help older people keep going to enjoy every day they are lucky enough to have. He does this writing books, creating instructional videos, and giving inspiring talks to groups of seniors. His current interests include reading and learning to write, to fight climate change and reduce animal and ecological suffering. He enjoys solving problems to help people in pain. Kevin is an avid Ironman-distance triathlete, vegetable gardener and vegan. Some of his work is designed to help people who like himself have aortic and other vascular diseases. He enjoys friends, family and not being dead for as long as possible.